FITNESS PROFESSIONALS

CIRCUIT TRAINING

a complete guide to planning and instructing
2nd edition

DEBBIE LAWRENCE AND BOB HOPE

A & C BLACK · LONDON

Thanks to Fitness Professionals Ltd (www.fitpro.com) for supporting the Fitness Professionals series

First published 2007 by
A&C Black Publishers Ltd
38 Soho Square, London W1D 3HB
www.acblack.com

ISBN 9780713683646

A CIP catalogue record for this book is available from the British Library.

Typeset in Berthold Baskerville Regular by Palimpsest Book Production Ltd, Grangemouth, Stirlingshire

Cover and inside photography © Grant Pritchard

Printed and bound in Great Britain by Biddles Ltd, Kings Lynn, Norfolk

This book is produced using paper that is made from wood grown in managed, sustainable forests. It is natural, renewable and recyclable. The logging and manufacturing processes conform to the environmental regulations of the country of origin.

CONTENTS

ACKNOWLEDGEMENTS

Being able to share my knowledge and experience to inspire and encourage others has always been, and continues to be, my dream. Writing a book is always a massive challenge and I am grateful that once again I have made the effort to fulfil my dreams and manage the challenge.

On a professional level, my thanks go to co-author Bob Hope. Thanks for using your valuable time to design so many wonderful, imaginative and creative circuits. I feel they give this book a really unique quality.

Also, thanks to Keith Smith from YMCA FIT for his special input to the older adults' circuit training chapter. Thanks for sharing the wealth of your experience and designing an excellent functional circuit for the older adult.

Thanks to the team of staff at A&C Black for being fabulous to work with on the second edition of this book (Robert, Alex, Ruth, Lucy).

Huge thanks to the volunteer models: Louise, Tony, Mandy, Aimee and Keely.

On a personal level, my greatest thanks and appreciation must go to my friends and family: my partner Joe, and my mum Mary – thanks for encouraging me to begin my career in fitness.

Debbie Lawrence

I would like to thank the following people for their encouragement and assistance during the writing of this book:

Debbie Lawrence, without whom this book would definitely not have been written or completed. A brilliant teacher, writer, and friend. Great job, Debbie.

Alan Newman and Lee Land at the Plymouth YMCA, Steve Plant from the Isle of Wight College, and Steve Platt from Plymouth. All like-minded circuit training teachers, for allowing me to bounce ideas off them.

Jason Colgan, for his input on basketball. Paul Bedford for his knowledge, help and assistance on cycling and being a mate.

To my family, my wife and soul mate, Jan, who has been my strength and supporter for the past 35 years, who I love very much; my daughter Natasha Anne Hope Whelan who brightens mine and everyone's day; her husband Dean and Jack the best Grandson in the world. In memory of my Mum and Dad.

Thank you everyone. For all Circuit trainers everywhere, this is for you. Enjoy!

Bob Hope

INTRODUCTION

Circuit training is often erroneously portrayed as an intensive and stressful form of exercise, with a drill sergeant-type in the middle of a circuit bellowing orders at weary recruits. While circuit training can be used as an advanced form of training, we aim to demonstrate that it is simply another method of training to develop fitness. Circuit training is a very versatile and adaptable mode of training that requires the performance of a series of carefully selected exercises. The exercises chosen can be used to develop a specific component of fitness, specific skills for a particular sport, or for the needs of a particular specialist population. They can also be adapted to suit a wide range of fitness levels and to build an individual's or a team's fitness level as they improve. Participants often enjoy circuit training more than other modes of training because they are able to easily monitor their progress and really see the results of their hard work. Ultimately, there are numerous ways of modifying a circuit training session, which adds variety and fun and helps to maintain interest and motivation, so that those taking part are more likely to adhere to the exercise programme and to enjoy it at the same time!

The aim of this book is to explore the benefits and techniques of circuit training. Now fully revised from the first edition with updated information and additional material, and with key exercises demonstrated by photographs, it will act as a resource for circuit training teachers and also as a reference for sports coaches who need access to creative circuit ideas designed specifically for their sport.

Part One provides a basic introduction to fitness: why fitness is important – both physical and mental; and how fitness can be improved through training – specifically through circuit training.

Part Two identifies the skills required to plan, lead and teach a circuit training session. It outlines the necessary safety considerations and explores different approaches to circuit training, discussing the advantages and disadvantages of each. The final chapters look at different programme formats and methods of progressing and adapting each to accommodate the needs of participants.

Part Three discusses and demonstrates appropriate activities for warming up and cooling down, along with appropriate activities, exercises and session structures to improve the main components of fitness.

Part Four provides detailed instructions on how to perform and instruct a range of exercises appropriate for outdoor circuit training, training for older adults, and circuits for specific sports.

WHY CIRCUIT TRAINING?

1

THE BENEFITS OF CIRCUIT TRAINING

1

What are the general benefits of circuit training?

Circuit training is a safe, effective and fun approach to exercising that can be enjoyed by a variety of people; it is attractive to men and women, younger and older age groups, sportspeople and the general population. It can be performed indoors and outdoors, and in water.

To fully understand the benefits of circuit training it is necessary to explore the components of physical fitness and discuss how each of these can be improved through participation in a progressive circuit training programme. The components that contribute to physical fitness are:

- cardiovascular fitness
- muscular strength
- muscular endurance
- flexibility
- motor fitness (includes agility, balance, reaction time, speed, power and co-ordination).

It is also necessary to discuss how to progress these fitness components and provide overload to the specific physiological systems. Therefore, the principles of training will also be discussed in relation to each component of fitness. Principles include:

- frequency (how often)
- intensity (how hard)

- time/duration (how long)
- type of training.

The contributions that circuit training makes to health and wellbeing will also be explored in relation to the following components, which are believed to encompass most aspects of total fitness/health:

- physical fitness
- social fitness
- mental fitness
- emotional fitness
- nutritional fitness
- medical fitness
- spiritual fitness.

This chapter therefore explores how participation in a progressive circuit training programme can contribute towards improving and developing our physical fitness and lead us towards the optimum of total fitness.

Aerobic and anaerobic

The body has to create energy to function both during times of rest and activity. This energy comes in the form of a chemical called Adenosine Tri Phosphate (ATP). ATP cannot be stored inside a muscle in large amounts, but is continually broken down to create energy and then reproduced inside the muscle via the body's energy systems (aerobic or anaerobic).

When resting and inactive, demands for energy and ATP production are lower. During exercise and activity, the demands for energy and ATP production are greater to enable muscle contraction and all the other physiological processes required by the exercising body.

The main factors that determine the energy system used to re-synthesise ATP are the:

- intensity of the activity
- duration of the activity
- fitness level of the person performing the activity
- skill level of the person performing the activity – that is, how familiar they are with performing that activity (specificity).

Generally speaking, activities which are of a **lower intensity** and can be continued for **longer durations** will use the **aerobic** energy system predominantly. This means the individual will be using oxygen to create energy. Activities that are of a **higher intensity** and can only be performed for **shorter durations** will use the **anaerobic** energy systems, which do not use oxygen to create energy. This means the individual would not be using oxygen to perform the activity and therefore would have to slow down or stop because the energy source had expired or a build-up of waste products (lactic acid, which causes the burn) would inhibit further work.

Realistically, during a circuit training session, all the energy systems will interweave to enable activities of different intensity to be performed. At different times throughout the workout, certain energy systems may be more predominant.

A basic introduction and summary of the body's energy systems is provided in Table 1.1. Readers wishing to study further are recommended to read other anatomy and physiology texts listed in the references.

Table 1.1	The body's energy systems		
Energy System	**Creatine Phosphate**	**Lactic Acid/ glycogen**	**Oxygen**
Anaerobic / aerobic	Anaerobic	Anaerobic	Aerobic
Fuel used	Creatine phosphate	Glycogen	Glycogen, fat (in the presence of glycogen), protein (sparingly). The latter is not ideal as a main fuel and would only be used in conditions where other fuels were unavailable
Fuel stored	Muscles	Muscles and liver	Glycogen stored in muscle Fat stored as adipose tissue

Table 1.1	The body's energy systems cont.		
			Protein not stored in same way. Excess protein intake stored as fat
Amounts of fuel	Limited – only a few available	Moderate supply – from a few seconds up to two to three minutes When broken down without oxygen, waste product lactic acid is produced	Moderate supply of glycogen, more plentiful supply of fat System can sustain activity for as long as fuel available
Intensity, duration and type of activity	High intensity Short duration 100m sprint Throwing and jumping events Strength training	Moderate to high intensity 400m sprint Anaerobic endurance – eight to 25 repetitions approximately	Low to moderate intensity Longer duration Marathon running Long distance swimming and cycling Circuit weight training
Waste products	Creatine – no harmful side effects. Cannot be used until resynthesised.	Lactic acid – inhibits muscle contraction. Burning sensation – intensity of activity needs to lower for work to continue.	Heat generated produces water. The body sweats to maintain a comfortable temperature Carbon dioxide – transported to lungs and exhaled

What is cardiovascular fitness?

Cardiovascular fitness is the ability of the heart, lungs and circulatory system to transport and utilise oxygen efficiently. It is sometimes referred to as cardio-respiratory fitness, stamina, or aerobic fitness.

Why do we need cardiovascular fitness?

We need a strong and efficient heart, respiratory and circulatory system to maintain our quality of life, to participate in sporting and recreational activities and to prevent the onset of circulatory diseases linked with inactivity (coronary heart disease and high blood pressure).

The long-term benefits of cardiovascular training

- Stronger heart muscle
- Increased stroke volume (amount of blood pumped in each contraction of the heart)
- Increased capillarisation (more blood vessels delivering blood and oxygen to the muscles)
- Increased mitochondria (cells in which aerobic energy is produced)
- Increased metabolic rate (rate at which we burn calories)
- More effective weight management
- More effective stress management
- Decreased body fat
- Decreased cholesterol levels
- Decreased blood pressure
- Decreased risk of coronary heart disease

How can we improve our cardiovascular fitness?

To improve the fitness of the heart, respiratory and circulatory system, we need to perform rhythmic activities which use the large muscles of the body. These should be performed on a regular basis, at a moderate intensity and for a prolonged duration. Adherence to this type of exercise programme will induce the necessary long-term health related improvements to the cardiovascular system. The recommended training requirements for improvements of cardiovascular fitness are outlined in Table 1.2.

What types of activity are appropriate in a circuit training session?

The most effective exercises for bringing about the desired training benefits and improving cardiovascular fitness in a circuit training session are those that require us to use the large muscles of the lower body. Any movement which shifts our body weight against the force of gravity in the following ways is effective:

- upwards (jumping and stepping)
- downwards (squatting and lunging)
- travel across (shuttle runs and gallops)

These are illustrated in Figure 1.1 on page 7.

Jumping activities require plenty of muscular effort to move our centre of gravity upwards, away from the ground. They also create greater momentum and demand that our muscles work harder to maintain correct alignment. A disadvantage of too many jumping (high-impact) movements is that greater stress will be placed on the joints. They should therefore be combined with other lower-impact activities to avoid causing injury. Lower-impact activities that elevate the centre of gravity upwards include exercises using a step or bench.

Table 1.2	Recommended training guidelines for cardiovascular fitness
Frequency How often should we perform these activities?	Three to five times a week Three times a week is sufficient for people exercising at higher intensities. More than three times a week is recommended for people exercising at low levels of intensity Rest days and vigorous training days should be alternate. Vary the activities and alter the impact to avoid injury to the muscles and joints NB: People with low fitness may follow Department of Health activity guidelines (see Table 1.3)
Intensity How hard should we be working?	55–90/65–90 per cent MHR A range of 70–85 per cent MHR is sufficient for most individuals to improve cardiovascular fitness when combined with appropriate frequency and duration Lower levels of intensity are appropriate for the less active. However, duration may need to be increased
Time/Duration How long should we sustain these activities for?	Training from between 20–60 minutes of continuous or intermittent activity e.g. accumulating 10-minute bouts throughout the day (see Department of Health guidelines in Table 1.3) Minimum duration to improve cardiovascular fitness in apparently healthy adults is 20–30 minutes. All durations exclude necessary time for warm up and cool down. Less fit groups will need to progress gradually to increased durations
Type/Mode/Specificity What types of activities are most effective?	Rhythmical, continuous activities that use large muscle groups e.g. walking, swimming, running, cycling, dancing, rowing, stepping

Adapted using ACSM Guidelines (2005)

Fig. 1.1

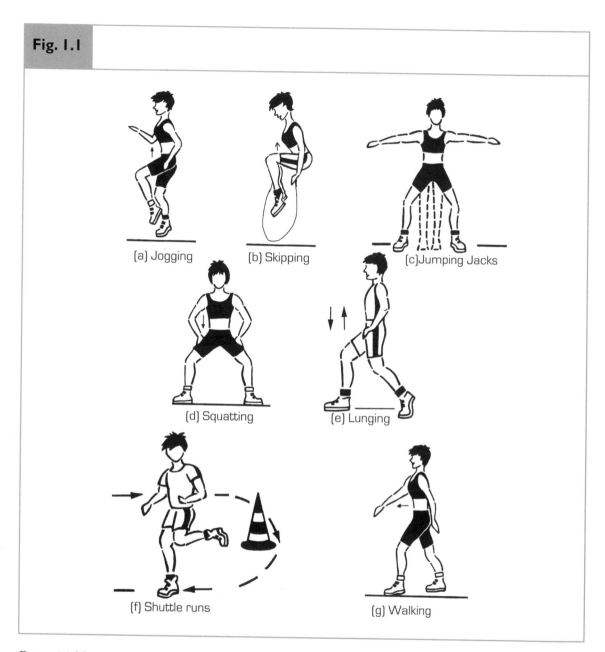

Figure 1.1 Movements of the centre of gravity during jumping, bending and travelling. Jogging, skipping or jumping movements lift the weight of the body and the centre of gravity upwards through a larger range of motion; squatting, lunging and other bending movements require the body weight and centre of gravity to be shifted downwards and then upwards against the force of gravity; travelling movements involve the work of more muscles and increase the range of motion through which the centre of gravity travels.

Other lower-impact moves include deep bending exercises such as squats and lunges. These utilise the larger muscles of the legs to bend and straighten the knee and hip joints, and transfer the weight of our body against the force of gravity. It is worth noting that excessive repetition of either stepping or deep bending movements can be equally stressful for the body if they are not alternated with other activities. Travelling movements shift the resistance of our body across the force of gravity. They require greater muscular effort and the recruitment of a larger number of muscles. Travelling movements which require us to move in many different directions are excellent for varying the stress placed on the weight-bearing joints, provided the direction and type of movements are varied. Movements of the upper body are comparatively less effective because the muscles in this region are smaller and make a relatively insignificant demand for oxygen. Arm movements above the head will elevate the heart rate because the heart has to work harder to pump blood upwards against gravity, though this may have an adverse affect on blood pressure.

Table 1.3	Targets for physical activity
Frequency	Work towards building activity into daily routine on five days of the week (minimum)
Intensity	Work at a moderate level where you feel mildly breathless, warm but comfortable (Level 3–4 on the adapted RPE intensity scale)
Time	Work towards performing the chosen activities for a total of **30 minutes**. This can be broken down and accumulated, for example: **3 x 10-minute** slots of activity each day **2 x 15-minute** slots of activity each day
Type	Any activity that fits well into your daily lifestyle! For example: • Walking to the station • Walking the kids to school • Vigorous housework • Cleaning the car • Walking up and down stairs more frequently • Dancing to a piece of music at home • Active hobbies • Structured exercise and sporting activities • A combination of activity, exercise and sport
	This recommendation can be tailored specifically to the lifestyle, preference and needs of the individual and is particularly relevant for people who find it easier and more acceptable to increase physical activity by incorporating it into their everyday life

From *Fitness Professionals – GP Referral Schemes*. Lawrence and Barnett (A&C Black: 2006)

Ultimately, a variety of movements for the larger leg muscles are safer and more effective. A variety of cardiovascular exercises are illustrated and explained in Chapter 9.

Individuals who are less fit can work towards developing their cardiovascular fitness by following the Department of Health (2005) recommendations for physical activity to maintain general health. These targets are outlined in Table 1.3. NB: These recommendations were established by the Department of Health (1996) and have been reiterated throughout all subsequent white papers produced by the Department of Health (2004 and 2005).

What is muscular strength and endurance (MSE)?

Muscular strength is the ability of our muscles to exert a near maximal force to lift a resistance. This is traditionally achieved by performing exercises that require us to lift heavy resistances for a short period of time (high resistance and low repetitions).

Muscular endurance requires a less maximal force to be exerted, but for the muscle contraction to be maintained for a longer duration. This requires a lighter resistance to be lifted for an extended period of time (low resistance and high repetitions).

Why do we need muscular strength and endurance?

Our muscles need to have strength and endurance for a number of reasons.

Our muscles work in pairs. If one of the pair is contracted or worked too frequently and becomes too strong, and the other is not worked sufficiently or is allowed to become weaker, then our joints will be pulled out of the correct alignment. This may cause injury or create postural defects such as rounded shoulders or excessive curvature of the spine. These defects are illustrated in Figure 1.2 on page 12.

Our muscles should therefore be kept sufficiently strong to maintain a correct posture. However, it may be that we have to specifically target certain muscles to compensate for the imbalances caused by our work and daily activities. For the majority of people with a sedentary lifestyle, it is worthwhile strengthening the abdominal muscles, the muscles between the shoulder blades (trapezius and rhomboids), and possibly the muscles of the back (erector spinae).

Long-term benefits of muscular and endurance training

- Increased bone density (more calcium laid down)
- Decreased risk of osteoporosis
- Improved posture and alignment
- Improved performance of sporting and recreational activities
- Efficient performance of daily tasks
- Improved body shape and tone
- Improved self-image
- Improved self-confidence
- Stronger muscles, ligaments and tendons which are more supportive to movement

Table 1.4	Recommended guidelines for training muscular strenth and endurance
Frequency How often should we perform these activities?	Two to three times per week (same muscle groups) for muscular fitness Alternate rest and training days (not consecutive days)
Intensity How hard should we be working?	To the point of near fatigue, while maintaining good technique For strength gains, lifting a weight equivalent to 75 per cent or above of one repetition maximum (most that can be lifted for one repetition) For endurance, lifting below 75 per cent of one repetition maximum
Time/Duration How long should we sustain these activities for?	For strength gains, lower repetitions with heavier resistance (up to eight repetitions) For endurance, higher repetitions with lower resistance (above 12 repetitions) For muscular fitness, work with a moderate resistance that can be lifted (8–12 repetitions) One set of 10–15 (moderate intensity) is recommended for older adults Training time will vary depending on the level of fitness, number of exercises, muscle groups and fitness goals
Type/Mode/Specificity What type of activities are most effective?	8–10 exercises targeting the main muscle groups Choose activities that are comfortable throughout the range of movement: • Free weights • Resistance machines • Body weight exercises • Body bars • Exercise bands

How can we improve our muscular strength and endurance?

Isolated exercises that focus on specific muscles/muscle groups are most effective. Weight training is a typical training mode, although callisthenic exercises, such as press-ups, sit-ups and squats, that require us to lift our body weight against gravity and manipulate the length of the body's leverage, can be equally effective. These activities need to be performed approximately two to three times a week for sufficient improvement to be made. The resistance lifted should promote a fatigued feeling in the muscle after anything between seven and 25 repetitions. The gains achieved by an individual will be determined by the number of repetitions they are able to perform. The recommended training requirements for improving muscular strength and muscular endurance are outlined in Table 1.3. A variety of MSE exercises are illustrated and explained in Chapter 10.

What is flexibility?

Flexibility is the ability of our joints and muscles to move through their full potential range of motion. It is sometimes referred to as suppleness or mobility.

Why do we need flexibility?

The ability of the joints and muscles to move through their full potential range of motion is essential for a number of reasons.

It should be recognised that if we participate in sporting activities we may require a little extra flexibility work for specific muscles. A needs analysis and flexibility focus for specific

sports is outlined in Chapter 16. However, for everyday purposes we should ensure that we are flexible enough to meet the demands placed on our body.

The long-term benfits of flexibility training

- Improved range of motion in the joints and muscles
- Improved posture and joint alignment giving the body a more slimline poise
- More economical movements and reduced unnecessary energy expenditure
- Enhanced performance of sporting and everyday activities
- Reduced tension in the muscles
- Reduced risk of injury when performing movements that require us to move quickly into extended positions, such as bending down, reaching up and away, and twisting around.

How can we improve our flexibility?

Flexibility can be maintained or improved (developed) by the frequent (daily) performance of activities which require our muscles and joints to move through their full range of motion. Since most lifestyles do not naturally provide these opportunities, stretching activities are incorporated into most fitness programmes. Stretching activities are those which require:

- the two ends of the muscle, the origin and insertion, to move further apart in a controlled manner
- the muscle to lengthen and relax.

Fig. 1.2   Curvatures of the spine

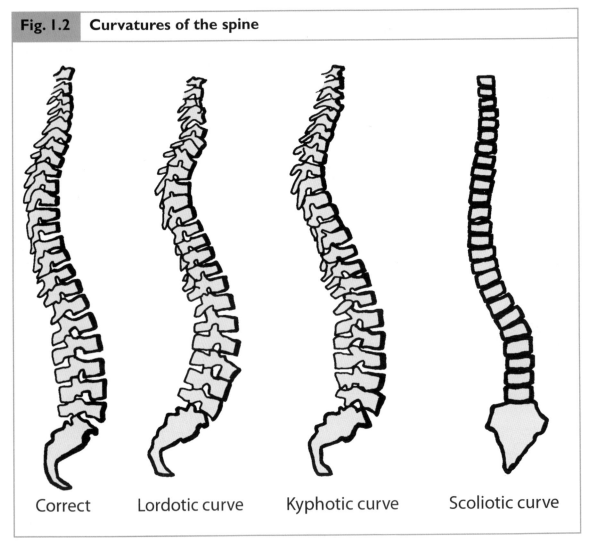

Correct   Lordotic curve   Kyphotic curve   Scoliotic curve

NB: Lordosis can be exaggerated during pregnancy when the abdominal muscles weaken and the weight of the baby can create a forward tilt of the pelvis.

Kyphosis can be caused by slumping over a desk all day, and also possibly by driving. The pectoral muscles become shorter and tighter and the trapezius and rhomboid muscles lengthen and weaken.

Scoliosis can be exaggerated by continuously carrying a bag of shopping using the same side of the body. The muscles on one side of the body would be stronger than those on the opposite side of the body.

Static stretch positions are generally advocated as safer. These require comfortable, supportive positions to be adopted and held for an appropriate duration. They enable the tension initially felt in the muscle (the stretch reflex) to dissipate (desensitisation) and allow the muscle to relax.

Ballistic stretches, or those which move too quickly or too far into the stretch position, may cause us to exceed our range of motion (overstretch), in which case the muscle will not relax. This is the main disadvantage of ballistic, bouncy movements. A further disadvantage is that they may potentially create muscle tearing and damage to the ligaments and other tissues which surround the joint. In the long term this may reduce the stability of the joints and create

hypermobility (laxity or looseness of the ligaments around the joints). Dynamic stretches, where the muscle is progressively moved to an extended range of motion, can be inducted for participants with higher levels of body awareness. Dynamic stretching involves controlled movement (not ballistic) that moves the muscle to the end of the range of motion and then back to the starting length/position. A few repetitions of the movement are performed to enable the muscle to lengthen progressively. For example, leg curls/hamstring curls (a knee mobility exercise) could be used as a dynamic lengthening for the quadriceps muscle. The hamstrings contract to raise the heel to the buttocks and the quadriceps (antagonist muscle) lengthens to allow the movement.

Table 1.5	Recommended guidelines for training flexibility
Frequency How often should we perform these activities?	A minimum of two to three times per week; ideally five to seven days a week The body must be warm prior to stretching to prevent muscle tearing and to enhance the range of motion
Intensity How hard should we be working?	Stretch positions should be taken to a point of mild tension, not discomfort, and held for an extended period of time Two to four repetitions can be performed for each stretch using the same or different stretch positions
Time/Duration How long should we sustain these activities for?	Hold static for 15 to 30 seconds
Type/Mode/Specificity What types of activity are most effective?	Static stretches are recommended for the general population.

Adapted using ACSM Guidelines (2005)

The recommended training requirements for improving our flexibility are outlined in Table 1.5. A variety of stretching exercises are illustrated and explained in Chapter 7.

When should we stretch in a circuit training session?

It is important to stretch the muscles at the end of the warm-up to prepare them for the main workout. Static stretches are appropriate for persons with low motor skills/body awareness. Dynamic stretches are appropriate for persons with higher levels of body awareness. It is also important to stretch the muscles after they have finished working to maintain their range of motion.

To improve flexibility, static developmental stretches must be included at the end of the programme. Developmental stretches involve the muscle being lengthened to the end of the range of motion, where a mild tension is felt (stretch reflex). When the tension in the muscle eases (desensitises), the stretch can then be taken further. At this point, the tension will reoccur in the muscle to prevent over-stretching. The tension should be allowed to ease off, and when it does the stretch can be held for a longer period of time. This process can be repeated a number of times, if desired. Once an appropriate and extended range of motion is achieved, the stretch should be held still for as long as is comfortable.

What is motor fitness?

Motor fitness is a skill-related component of fitness and refers to a number of inter-related factors, including agility, balance, speed, coordination, reaction time and power.

Why do we need motor fitness?

Motor fitness requires the effective transmission and management of messages and responses between the central nervous system (the brain and spinal cord) and the peripheral nervous system (sensory and motor). The peripheral nervous system collects information via the sensory system; the central nervous system receives and processes this information and sends an appropriate response via the motor system, which initiates the appropriate response.

Motor fitness is perhaps more applicable to the sportsperson, but it can have an indirect effect on the improvement of our fitness in the other health-related fitness components. For example, learning to perform movements such as squats with correct posture and alignment will make them more effective and efficient. If we move skilfully and accurately we can improve the effectiveness of the activities we perform. In addition, by learning to perform exercises with the correct technique, we will reduce the risk of injury that can be caused by moving with our body in poor alignment. Therefore, improved motor fitness will maximise both the safety and effectiveness of our performance.

How do we improve our motor fitness?

Managing our body weight, manoeuvring our centre of gravity, coordinating our body movements, moving at different speeds, in different directions and at different intensities, will all contribute to improving our motor fitness in the long term. If we want to improve our motor fitness, we must specifically and repeatedly train the aspect we wish to improve. The use of explosive movements may emphasise the development of power, while shuttle runs may develop speed. In addition, the use of a number or whistle blow to dictate a specific movement to be performed may develop reaction time in addition to other skill-related components.

If we want to perform a quick, co-ordinated sequence of movements (a golf swing, a dance routine, a discus or javelin throw), then we need to perform the specific movements that make up that sequence. However, we may need to train ourselves to develop the necessary skills, which in these examples are speed, power and accurate co-ordination. Therefore, we should break down the sequence into smaller components and perform each component in isolation and at a slower pace. By progressively linking one component to another, and moving at a quicker pace, we will, in time, develop the necessary skills to perform the whole sequence at the appropriate speed. We will have therefore improved our motor fitness.

However, if we then wish to learn to walk the tightrope, we need to develop different skills in a different way. Balance will be a very important skill for this activity. But performing our co-ordinated sequence of movements will not assist our balance on the tightrope. Training to improve our motor fitness must therefore specifically relate to the activities we need or want to perform. However, we must ensure that we are not put off if we cannot initially do something. In time, we can all learn the necessary skills to perform any activity. The key is to break down the skill and allow ourselves the time to develop it slowly. A good teacher will break down the skill for us, and encourage us as we practise and develop.

If the development of motor fitness is a specific intention of the workout, the requirements and needs of the participants should be analysed. Chapters 9 and 16 are devoted to discussing, illustrating and outlining a needs analysis with example plans for different sporting activities.

Summary of the benefits of physical fitness

Regular performance of each of the activities described will significantly improve physical fitness and bring about the improvements specified throughout. By improving our physical fitness we are making endless contributions to enhancing our quality of life and improving our overall health.

Factors affecting physical fitness

A number of factors will affect and contribute to an individual's physical fitness, and sometimes fitness potential. Sports coaches and teachers need to be aware of these and recognise how they will affect an individual's participation in a circuit training session. Sports coaches also need to be able to adapt exercises and make recommendations to their clients regarding some of these factors.

Heredity

The genetic make-up of an individual will to some extent determine how his or her body responds to a programme of activities: 75% of our potential is inherited, while 25% is changeable. It could therefore be assumed that if an individual's birth parents were athletic, they too would share those genes, and thus have greater potential to develop their athletic ability.

Body type

A further consideration is the individual's body type. This is closely linked to heredity and is determined genetically. Their 'morphic' type

Fig. 1.3	Different body types: mesomorph (left), endomorph (centre), ectomorph (right)

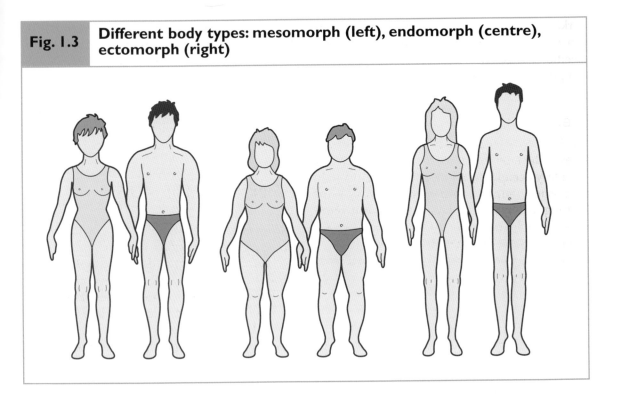

will also influence their physical capability. The characteristics of the three main body types are illustrated in Figure 1.3.

Ectomorphs tend to be leaner, with a lower proportion of body fat and muscle. They also have narrower shoulders and hips and tend to appear taller. They will generally favour long-distance running events. Their low muscle mass and longer levers will affect their ability to lift heavier weights.

Endomorphs tend to have a more rounded appearance. They have a higher proportion of body fat, which tends to be stored around the middle of the body (around the abdomen for men, and around the hips for women). The extra weight will mean that they find long-distance events tough. In addition, running events and impact exercises will be more stressful to their joints, which are already

carrying more weight. The higher proportion of body fat will mean that they float with more ease. They may therefore find water-based activities easier than either an ectomorph or mesomorph would. This is because body fat assists floatation and maintains a comfortable body temperature.

Mesomorphs tend to have a more athletic appearance. They have broader shoulders, narrower hips and a higher proportion of muscle mass. This body type lends itself to strength training and bodybuilding.

Age

Our potential to improve fitness declines with age. However, the speed of decline can be reduced through regular exercise and activity. Specific considerations need to be made when working with older adults (Chapter 14), and also younger children and teenagers, because specific changes occur to the body's anatomy and physiology throughout the life span.

Lifestyle

The lifestyle of an individual will also affect their fitness. The fitness and health of a person with a sedentary occupation and lifestyle will be greatly diminished, while a person who engages in sporting activities or a person who has a more active lifestyle (housework, DIY, gardening) and regularly undertakes activities that require a moderate degree of physical effort will maintain a reasonable level of fitness.

Health

A person's state of health will affect their fitness and their participation in physical activities. Injuries, hypertension, asthma and diabetes are but a few of the conditions that need to be identified. Coaches and teachers should undertake a thorough health screening of all individuals prior to their participation in a circuit training programme. Participants will then need to be either referred to their GP or have their needs accommodated within the programme. Further information on health screening is provided in Chapter 3. Those who wish to know more about specific medical conditions are advised to refer to a family health encyclopaedia or visit their GP. Information regarding working with clients referred to exercise by their GP is provided in *Fitness Professionals – GP Referral Schemes.* Lawrence and Barnett (A&C Black: 2006).

Individuals' goals

This is not so much a factor affecting fitness as a further consideration for circuit training teachers. Some information regarding what the client(s) want to achieve will influence the design, structure and choice of exercises selected for performance within the circuit. For example, a person who is attending to improve their general health and fitness will have different wants and needs than a sports person or an older adult. Guidelines for working with different needs are provided in Part Four.

What is total fitness?

Total fitness requires us to be socially, mentally, emotionally, nutritionally and medically fit, as well as physically fit. It demands that we pay attention to our lifestyle, our diet, our stress levels, our emotions, our ability to communicate, our need to relax and recuperate, as well as our physical fitness. Circuit training is one of many effective modes of improving the components of total fitness.

What is social fitness and how can it be improved?

Social fitness involves interaction and communication with people. Circuit training is a group activity and often involves some partner work, team activities and other group activities, which lighten the atmosphere, encourage interaction and potentially enhance social fitness.

What is mental and emotional fitness, and how can it be improved?

Mental and emotional fitness refers to our psychological wellbeing. The pressures of daily life can have a negative effect on our mental and emotional fitness, causing us to feel tired, anxious and stressed. Stress is a contributory factor to coronary heart disease. It therefore needs to be managed and any negative effects reduced.

There are a number of reasons why regular circuit training can help with stress management. Firstly, the physical exertion necessary to perform exercises provides us with an excellent way of releasing the pressure and tension that builds up. Secondly, when we take part in aerobic exercise, we increase the circulation of endorphins, a hormone which gives us an enhanced feeling of wellbeing. This feeling can last for much longer than the duration of the actual exercise session. Thirdly, the socialisation process can affirm our self-worth and sense of belonging. Finally, the long-term improvements to our body shape and physical appearance can enhance self-esteem, self-image and self-confidence.

The stretching exercises at the end of the session can also have a relaxing effect on the mind and body. As the body slows down, the mind can also be encouraged to slow down, providing a great relief from the ever-increasing pace of daily living.

What is nutritional fitness and how can we improve it?

Nutritional fitness requires us to eat a balanced diet that sustains our energy levels and promotes improved health. It is therefore essential that we eat a balanced diet from the main food groups:

• carbohydrates (pasta, potatoes, bread)
• fats (cheese, milk, butter)
• proteins (beans, pulses, meat)
• vitamins and minerals (vegetables and fruit)
• water.

We should also ensure that the quantity of food we consume is appropriate to meet our requirements.

Some general guidelines for improving our diet include:

• eat less saturated fat
• eat less sugar
• eat less salt
• eat more complex carbohydrates*
• eat more fruit and vegetables ('five a day')
• eat sufficient fibre
• maintain a sufficient calorie intake
• drink more water.

*i.e. bread, rice, pasta etc., which are slower to digest, serve as a more effective energy source and assist with regulating blood sugar levels.

What is medical fitness and how can we improve it?

Medical fitness is our state of health and requires the body to be in an optimal working order. Most recent government white papers report on the declining health of the nation and the role that exercise and activity can play in managing and preventing some conditions, such as osteoporosis, stress and depression, high blood cholesterol, high blood pressure, obesity, coronary heart disease and so on.

Regular exercise, activity and improved fitness can encourage us to eat more healthily, maintain a healthy body composition and manage stress more effectively. It can also build social networks and relationships, which in turn may encourage us to cut down or remove habits that have an adverse affect on our health, such as smoking, drinking excessive alcohol or eating too much of the less nutritious foods, all of which contribute to increasing health risk.

A well-structured and effectively taught circuit training programme has the potential to bring about all the necessary improvements in physical and total fitness. Later chapters in this book discuss how to structure the session to maximise these benefits for the variety of individuals who might attend.

What is spiritual fitness and how can we improve it?

Spiritual fitness reflects our view and vision of the world (inner and outer), which can be influenced by belief systems, attitudes and values passed down through generations within families, schools, societies, cultures and religions.

From a spiritual perspective, each of us is a unique individual with our own life journey and our own life lessons. We each make choices to follow a different life path and we each have the potential to choose how we respond and grow from life's challenges, whether they be:

- medical (our health)
- physical (our fitness and appearance)
- nutritional (eating behaviour and diet)
- social (our relationships, our habits, the prejudices we may experience or hold)
- mental (whether our outlook is positive or negative)
- emotional – how we respond to life events which all contribute to the person we become.

Spiritual growth is a lifelong journey! It is about awareness, mindfulness, responsiveness and wholeness. Yoga and tai chi are specific methods of exercise which emphasise a more spiritual connection. They aim to unite the mind, body and spirit by focusing attention on breathing, performance of specific movements and postures, awareness of the flow of energy and the personal experience the individual has within the session. However, other forms of exercise are equally accessible and can offer an equally valid method for focusing this awareness back to the self and the body and away from external triggers which can create disharmony and imbalance in all the areas listed above. For some a quiet walk in the park provides them with this access; for others a more active circuit session offers that focus.

Summary of the benefits of circuit training

Circuit training will potentially:
- improve all components of physical fitness
- assist improvement of skill-related components of fitness essential for participation in sport
- assist with weight management
- promote social interaction
- encourage a healthier lifestyle
- assist with stress management
- improve self-esteem and confidence in physical appearance
- enhance feelings of wellbeing
- improve overall health.

PLANNING AND TEACHING A CIRCUIT TRAINING PROGRAMME

PART TWO

Circuit training involves far more than linking together a sequence of exercises and shouting directions at a group of people. It requires an awareness of:

- the necessary teaching skills and qualities to deliver a safe and effective session
- the health and safety considerations that need to be thought through in the planning stage, prior to delivering the circuit
- individual abilities and needs and knowledge of how to accommodate these throughout the session (see also Part Four)
- how to progress and adapt specific exercises (see also Part Three)
- how to vary the programme to maintain creativity and participant interest.

This section of the book explores each of these aspects in the following chapters.

TEACHER QUALITIES AND SKILLS

What are the qualities of a good teacher?

A good teacher should always be friendly, approachable and show concern for the health and safety of participants. He or she should be patient, motivating and encouraging, interested in participants, willing to listen, humorous and sensitive to participants' needs. The list of qualities is endless.

What are the roles of the teacher?

Planning and preparation

All activities should be prepared and planned in advance with regard given to the group, the environment and the equipment available. The teacher should arrive early to the session to make any last-minute safety checks and adjustments. They should be competent and equipped to adapt their planned session, should this prove necessary. For example, if the room is cold, or if more people arrive than planned for, they should be able to alter the routine accordingly.

At the start of the session they should always introduce themselves to new participants and encourage individuals to communicate their personal fitness goals and any special requirements. They should be confident and sufficiently knowledgeable to deal with any special requirements. Should they not be

qualified to deal with a special need, they should know whom to refer participants to, for example a doctor.

Teaching

The teacher will need to maintain control of the class before, during and after the session. Control should be maintained throughout the session by giving clear and accurate instructions and demonstrations, and advance cueing of each activity. They should also be vigilant, and monitor class performance at all times, giving coaching advice on an individual basis. In addition, they should encourage the class when they perform an exercise particularly well. If a participant is struggling they should be able to adapt the exercise for them.

How can the teacher communicate effectively throughout the session?

The primary aim of the coach is to communicate with the class. Participants need to know:

- what exercise they should be doing (instructions)
- when they should be doing it (cueing)
- how they should be doing it (safety points) and, if they cannot do it, they need to be shown

- how to adapt the exercise to meet their needs (alternatives).

There are two ways of communicating this information: 1. **visually** – demonstrations and body language; 2. **verbally** – spoken instructions.

The combined usage of visual and verbal communication strategies is usually the most effective as people learn in different ways. To slavishly adopt one single strategy over another can reduce one's effectiveness as a teacher. However, there are further issues to consider.

How will voice volume and intonation affect communication?

Verbal communication requires the voice to be loud and clear. A voice that is too quiet will not be heard, especially outside or in a large sports hall where acoustics are notoriously bad. It may also infer that the coach is timid and lacks confidence. Alternatively, shouting will distort the sound of the voice and can make the teacher appear aggressive. Therefore, it is necessary to find a way of modulating the voice so that it is both audible and establishes control.

The intonation of the voice is also important. Monotone voices can become uninteresting, and will provide no emphasis to key coaching points. Voice intonation should be varied to emphasise key instructions and safety advice being given, and to reflect the atmosphere of the specific component of the session. It should be used to encourage in components of the class where participants are required to work harder (i.e. the main circuit), and should be softer during relaxation and stretching time.

How will the clarity of instruction affect communication?

Instructions need to be spoken at an appropriate pace and in a concise and precise manner to maximise their effectiveness. If instructions are rushed, they may seem garbled and will more than likely be misunderstood. Additionally, the vocabulary used should be recognisable by participants. If they do not know the names of the exercises they are supposed to perform they will not follow effectively. However, lengthy explanations will be tedious and participants will lose interest. This is when it is most useful to use visual coaching strategies.

How will visual cueing enhance communication?

Visual cues are gestures of the body. Gesturing with the arms can indicate the direction of movement. Gesturing with the fingers and hand can be used to show how many times the exercise should be performed, to cue a new move, or indicate a turn in the movement. Facial expressions can be used to encourage the class (smiling). All of these can assist immensely with class control and motivation.

However, too many gestures may become irritating and be hard to follow. In addition, the gestures used need to be consistent so that the class know what is expected of them. If visual cues are used, they need to be strong and clear. Small and weak visual signals do not provide effective control.

NB: an outline of some appropriate visual cues is listed in *The Complete Guide to Exercise to Music,* Debbie Lawrence (A&C Black: 2004).

However, it is advisable that teachers select and develop their own cues to assist with group management.

How can the circuit stations be introduced and controlled?

Teachers who are dealing with groups of participants will need to plan carefully to ensure adequate control is achieved. Participants will need to be introduced to the exercises performed at each exercise station. If they are not, they may be unsure of how to perform the exercises correctly.

There are two ways to remember the sequences of information that need to be given when introducing circuit activities to individuals. These are:
• N.A.M.S.E.T.
• I.D.E.A.

Both sequences provide a logical structure and order for giving information to circuit participants. However, they do not have to be used rigidly. For example, it may be appropriate for the teacher to demonstrate and explain the exercise first and then name the muscles and area working while the participants are performing.

Some teachers introduce stations after the re-warmer (see Chapter 13). However, this approach often lowers the intensity, unless participants are kept sufficiently active while the exercises are being demonstrated and explained. A more appropriate method of introducing the exercise stations is to perform each exercise at a lower intensity during the warm-up. This will assist with a progressive rise in intensity, maintain interest and improve the continuity and flow of the session.

Unfortunately, participants may still forget stations when the main circuit is in operation. The use of printed circuit training cards to illustrate the exercise to be performed at each station can act as a reminder. However, the diagrams need to be large and visible, and the written instructions clear. It is also useful if key coaching points are listed as safety reminders.

N	Name the exercise	Bicep curl
A	Name the area of the body targeted	Front of upper arm
M	Name the muscles working	Biceps
S E	Show and Explain the exercise	Demonstrate the exercise from different angles and give key teaching points
T	Teach the individual through exercise	Talk the individuals into the start position Talk them through performing the exercise by giving coaching points and observing and correcting technique Ask questions to see how individuals feel Offer alternatives when needed Talk them out of the exercise

I	Introduce the exercise Name the body and muscles working	Bicep curl Front of upper arm Biceps
D E	Demonstrate the exercise Explain the exercise	Demonstrate the exercise from different angles and give key teaching points
A	Activity	Talk the individuals into the start position Talk them through performing the exercise by giving coaching points and observing and correcting technique Ask questions to see how individuals feel Offer alternatives when needed Talk them out of the exercise

The use of assistant coaches and spotters may also help with effective control. However, they will need to be instructed carefully about their role and responsibilities. In reality, assistants are not frequently accessible. Therefore, if dealing with inexperienced groups without assistance, it is often easier to reduce the number of stations. Chapters 8 and 10 discuss different circuit training formats.

How can demonstrations be used to improve class performance?

A swift demonstration of a movement allows the coach to show exactly how the body should move and in which direction. However, it is essential that their body alignment and exercise technique are precise and accurate. A poor demonstration will be ineffective, since participants will have to interpret the exercise in their own way and may subsequently perform unsafely or ineffectively.

For very complex movements or those which require the use of equipment, it is advisable to demonstrate and allow participants to perform a dry run to check they can perform the movement prior to its inclusion in the circuit. However, the class should be kept moving to keep them warm and maintain the intensity of the workout. A movement that replicates the actual circuit station without using the equipment is most appropriate. For example: a power squat using the step can be performed without a step in the re-warmer, or a station using weights can be performed without weights to familiarise participants with the correct alignment for the exercise, while the teacher demonstrates using equipment.

Where should the teacher be positioned to demonstrate, observe and correct performance?

The teacher should be in a position where they can see and be seen by all participants. This will vary depending on the circuit layout. If the participants are all facing the same way it is best for the teacher to be in front and easily observed by all. If the participants are scatterered around, it is not so easy. During the circuit it is more effective for the teacher to be positioned outside of the circuit so that they can look inwards and move around to people who need specific help. It is recommended that the teacher circulates around the circuit to identify where corrections and further help are necessary.

Ending the session

At the end of the session, the coach should thank participants for attending, encourage them to leave in a quiet manner and invite questions. Any equipment used should be packed away safely. They should therefore be prepared to stay slightly later and longer than the scheduled duration of the class.

Evaluation

Once the session is complete, a good teacher will reflect on the class they have taught and evaluate their own practice and the class performance. Some questions an instructor can ask themselves to reflect on performance include:

• Were the planned components safe and effective?
• Could everyone cope with the activities?
• Were the participants able to follow demonstrations?
• Did they (the teacher) manage to observe and correct performance?

Evaluating one's performance is a very difficult skill to develop, however. It is therefore useful to seek further feedback from participants, employers and other teachers. Selecting another teacher to act as a critical friend can be an excellent way of developing one's ability to evaluate. The views of a knowledgeable other person allow you to reflect more deeply and see things from a different perspective, but you do need to pick a teacher who will tell you their honest, objective opinion.

HEALTH AND SAFETY IN THE CIRCUIT TRAINING ENVIRONMENT

3

Who can attend a circuit training session?

Everyone can benefit from attending a circuit training session. Indeed, most people can quite easily be accommodated within a session, provided alternatives are offered to meet any special requirements. However, some circuit programmes are quite high intensity and do not cater for specific requirements. Older adults

Health screening checks

It is advisable to check with a doctor and seek their consent prior to commencing any physical activity if you:

- have high blood pressure or heart disease, or cardiovascular or respiratory problems
- have suffered from chest pains, especially if they are associated with light activity requiring minimal effort
- are prone to headaches, fainting or dizziness
- are pregnant or have recently been pregnant
- have, or are recovering from, a joint problem or injury which may be aggravated by physical activity
- are taking medication or have any other medical condition
- have recently been ill
- are unused to exercise and over 35 years of age.

and ante-natal or post-natal women are two groups that are best advised to join a more specialist circuit training session rather than a general session. Training needs of older adults are discussed in Part Four. In addition, some participants will need to obtain permission from their doctor before embarking on any programme of physical activity. This is to ensure that the exercise programme will be appropriate to their needs and that they will not be placing their wellbeing at risk by participating in the session. They too are best advised to attend a more specialist or lower-level class once permission is granted. Teachers should advise participants who answer yes to any of the health screening checks outlined in Table 3.1 to check with their doctor prior to taking part in any physical activity.

How can the teacher gather information for health screening?

There are three methods of gaining information from and about the target group:

- Visual – things you can observe, e. g. gender, age, body shape and size
- Verbal – things you need to ask and be told by the participant
- Written – questionnaires.

A few of the advantages and disadvantages of the different screening methods are outlined in Table 3.1 on page 29.

Identifying the fitness goals and current health of individuals is only the first step in designing an appropriate circuit training programme. It is also necessary to take into account the working environment, the equipment being used in the session, and the clothing worn by participants. It is unsafe and ineffective to design a programme without identifying the peculiarities of different working environments. It is also unsafe and ineffective to design a programme using equipment without understanding how the equipment should be lifted and manoeuvred.

What are the main environmental considerations?

Space

The size and shape of the working environment will determine how many participants can take part and how many stations can be used, the amount of travelling moves and even the positioning of the teacher. Ideally, participants should be able to stand in one place, outstretch their arms in all directions and not come into contact with another person. If participants are able to reach another person, then the working area is probably overcrowded. This will make it difficult and potentially unsafe to use a large number of exercise stations and travelling movements and make it less safe to use equipment. It will also be difficult for the teacher to move around and correct movements. In a small space, it is always advisable to limit class numbers and provide additional sessions so that all participants can exercise safely and can be observed by the teacher.

In a large area, such as a sports field, maintaining control of the group is a major safety concern. The group needs to be managed so that the teacher can observe all participants carefully. Exercise stations and activities should not be spread so far apart as to render observation impossible. In larger areas and with larger groups it is advisable to use helpers and spotters to assist with group management.

An ideal environment is a wide, rectangular space, such as one section of a sports hall. This will allow for plenty of forward, sideways and circular travelling moves which will alter stress on the body. It will also allow for the circuit stations to be spread a safe distance apart, with enough room to move around equipment. In addition, it will provide plenty of space for the teacher to move around in.

Long, narrow rooms will require forward travelling movements to be reduced, and if there are a lot of people in the room, sideways travelling moves may also be limited. It will also make circular running moves more cramped along the short sides of the room. In addition, the teacher will need to vary their position frequently to see all participants. Adopting one position throughout the session will limit observation and prevent the teacher from making essential corrections to participants' performance. In this situation it is advisable for the teacher to use a variety of group organisation methods, which include facing the same direction, facing inwards in a circle, and moving around in a circle. This will enable them to maximise observation of the group as a whole and of individual participants.

Floor surface

Ideally, the floor should be sprung so that impact forces are minimised. Performing high-impact exercises on a solid floor (concrete) are contra-indicated because the movements will

Table 3.1	Advantages and disadvantages of different methods of screening	
Method of screening	**Advantages**	**Disadvantages**
Visual	• Quick • Can identify personal issues without asking questions which may cause embarrassment	• Cannot identify all medical conditions visually
Verbal	• Response is immediate • Information is up to date • Personal contact • Can probe and seek further information if necessary • Can highlight the importance of receiving the information • Can clarify and respond to questions asked	• Participants may be unwilling to provide personal information • Responses may not be totally truthful • There is no written record or proof of what has been asked, nor the response provided • Information provided may be forgotten • Time-consuming, since only one person can be spoken to at a time • Confidentiality – information should be obtained in private
Written	• Permanent record of questions asked and responses provided • If the questionnaire used provides a yes or no response, concerns can be identified relatively quickly • Can screen more than one person at a time	• Circumstances change, therefore requires regular updating • Screening forms need to be stored in a secure place and remain confidential • Questionnaires should be worded carefully to obtain an accurate response • Information requested needs to encourage a concise response (yes or no). Wordy responses may be difficult to interpret and will take longer to read • Reading responses to questionnaires is time-consuming

Adapted from *The Complete Guide to Exercise to Music*, Debbie Lawrence (A&C Black: 2004)

not be cushioned. This may cause jarring and injury to the joints, and shin splints.

If the floor surface is not sprung then the cardiovascular exercises selected should be predominantly low impact. This will avoid placing the joints under too much stress.

Alternatively, the session could be designed to feature more muscular strength and endurance work than cardiovascular work. It is better to adapt the session rather than limit opportunities for people to improve their fitness.

It is also essential to make sure that the floor

surface is cleaned regularly, without being so highly polished that it becomes slippery.

When working outside on a sports field, the teacher needs to be aware of the terrain for the same reasons stated above. They need to be aware if the surface is muddy and slippery, and where the surface is harder so that they can avoid inappropriate exercises. Furthermore, they must know where there are potholes or changes in the level of the surface. It is easy to twist and sprain an ankle joint if running or moving on uneven terrain.

A further consideration when working outside is the slope of the land. Continuous work on an uphill slope is very intense. Participants will fatigue quickly. Alternatively, a lot of work downhill will increase the amount of eccentric muscle work. This will increase the risk of delayed onset muscle soreness. Ideally, a variety of work uphill and downhill combined with some work on the flat will minimise these risks and provide a more balanced workout.

Temperature

It is potentially unsafe and ineffective to perform a very static stretch component in a cold environment. It is also unsafe and ineffective to perform a very high-intensity cardiovascular workout in an excessively hot environment. Therefore the type of session provided will need to be adapted. General guidelines are outlined in Table 3.2.

Safety considerations regarding equipment used in a circuit training session

There is a wide variety of equipment that can be used in a circuit training session. Benches, steps, pull-up bars, barbells, dumbbells, mats, bands, skipping ropes, cones and medicine balls are just a few. Equipment will add variety to the session and is an excellent method of progressing certain exercise stations.

When using equipment, the teacher should familiarise themselves with the specific manufacturer's guidelines to ensure that they use the equipment safely and effectively throughout the session. It may also be necessary for them to undertake further training to ensure that they are fully competent to operate the equipment safely.

When warming up prior to the circuit, the teacher must ensure that participants are fully aware of where equipment is positioned. Participants should be advised to move around carefully and avoid treading on different pieces of equipment. It is also essential for the exercise stations to be a safe distance apart so that there is enough space to perform the exercise and lift and lower equipment safely and effectively. Participants should also be encouraged to place dumbbells and barbells securely when they have finished using them, so that they do not roll across the floor and interfere with the work of others.

Stacking, storage and maintenance of equipment

All equipment should be stored and stacked safely. Again, the manufacturers' guidelines should be referred to. The following are recommended as general safety considerations:

- Store barbells, dumbbells, ropes, and bands in a large chest or in individual containers in the corner of the room
- Ensure that all equipment is lifted correctly
- Ensure steps are not stacked too high, and ideally are caged to prevent them from falling and sliding across the room when it is being used for other activities

Table 3.2	Adaptations for different environmental temperatures
Adaptations for a cold environment	**Adaptations for a hot environment**
Longer and more active warm-up	Shorter and less intense warm-up
More pulse-raising moves between stretches	Safer to perform more static stretches
Can include longer and more intense cardiovascular activities	Less intense and perhaps slightly shorter duration of cardiovascular activities
Perhaps spend less time on muscular strength and endurance activities. Too many stations in sequence may have a cooling effect on the body. It may therefore be advisable to alternate cardiovascular and muscular strength and endurance stations	Can spend more time working on muscular strength and endurance at specific stations. This can replace the decreased amount of higher intensity cardiovascular work
Shorter post-workout stretch. Perhaps combine stretches to save time and leave out or prioritise developmental stretches (perform maintenance stretches instead). Performing maintenance stretches at the end of the pulselower will assist in maintaining a comfortable working temperature	Can spend longer on post-workout stretches. Include more developmental stretches and hold for longer
Leave out relaxation techniques	Longer relaxation component
Longer, more active remobilisation. Perhaps keeping moving between stretches	Short remobilise
Wear appropriate warm clothing and remove layers progressively when warm. Apply layers of clothing as cooling down commences	Wearing cool, lightweight clothing will be essential. If working outside on a sunny day, use sunscreen to protect the skin from sunburn

NB: the adaptations suggested above will also be determined by the fitness of the group. The intensity and activities selected should also reflect the capabilities of the participants

- Ensure that wires from electrical equipment are not trailing across the floor and that all plug fittings are secure
- Stack exercise mats and benches neatly at the side or back of the room. Ensure they are cleaned regularly and replaced or maintained when necessary
- Check the condition of weights and bands regularly to ensure that all fixtures and fittings are secure
- When equipment is in use ensure that it is spaced out safely (i.e. ensure stations are not too close together).

Lifting equipment

When moving equipment in a circuit training session the teacher should ensure that all participants utilise the correct lifting technique – the dead-lift. This technique is explained and illustrated in Chapter 11.

Safety considerations regarding clothing worn in a circuit training session

Footwear

There is a whole range of different footwear available for exercise and fitness activities. Most sports companies design specific footwear for individual sports and activities. Therefore, participants should seek advice from either the sales staff in a sports shop or from the manufacturer before deciding on the most appropriate type. As a guideline, the footwear selected should be well-fitting, supportive and designed specifically for the type of activity for which it is to be used. Participants who take part in a number of different activities are probably wiser to invest in cross trainers which are designed for use in a variety of sports. In addition, exercisers should replace their footwear regularly. Constant use creates wear and tear on the shoes and they become less supportive. Ideally, footwear should be used exclusively for sporting activities and not for everyday use; this will increase the longevity of their service.

A further consideration for coaches and participants is to ensure that shoelaces are tied securely prior to commencing a workout.

Clothing

All clothing should be appropriately fitted, but not so tight that it restricts movement. The disadvantage of wearing baggy clothing is that it restricts observation of joint alignment, which makes it difficult for the teacher to correct technique. However, some participants may prefer to wear a T-shirt and tracksuit bottoms, as opposed to fitted cycling shorts, or leggings and T-shirt. If this is their preference then it should be accommodated. The main consideration is that the teacher should wear clothing that allows their body alignment to be fully visible, since participants will be required to follow the teacher's movements. Plastic trousers should not be worn when performing high-intensity activities, as they prevent the body from cooling down and may potentially cause overheating and fainting.

Jewellery and body piercings

All large items of jewellery such as rings, bracelets, bangles, earrings and necklaces should be removed before taking part in any physical activity. They may cause accidental injury to another participant and may become damaged or scratched during floor work or when using hand weights.

A further consideration is for participants who have body piercings. In particular, belly button rings and studs can catch on mats and other equipment and cause injury. Tongue rings are also a risk, as they can come loose during the workout and may be swallowed.

Eating and chewing gum

Never eat or chew gum during exercise, as it is easy for food to become lodged in the throat and block the airway and/or cause choking.

Summary

The safety considerations discussed in this chapter are only a few of the many issues which need to be considered prior to planning a circuit training session. Each sports facility will have its own rules and regulations (health and safety policy document) which teachers will need to adhere to and convey clearly to the class participants. It is therefore essential that the teacher becomes familiar with the requirements for the centre in which they teach. Combined efforts from all persons will ensure that the sessions programmed are safe, effective and comply with all current health and safety legislation.

APPROACHES TO DESIGNING AND MANAGING A CIRCUIT TRAINING SESSION

4

There are many different ways of managing and designing a circuit training programme. These include:

- the timing or method of controlling movement from one station to the next within the circuit
- the shape, layout and arrangement of the circuit stations
- the choice of exercises selected for completion at each of the stations. An outline of appropriate exercises to improve general fitness and for sport-specific training are provided in Parts 3 and 4 of this book.

The approach selected will be dependent on a number of factors. These include: fitness level, age, ability and requirements of the participants, i.e. general fitness or sport-specific training, class numbers, space, environmental conditions, and equipment and resources available. This chapter provides a basic introduction to some of the different approaches and explores the advantages and disadvantages of each.

Managing work time at each station

The time spent working on a specific station or exercise can be dictated by either timing each exercise, or specifying the number of repetitions to be performed. Both will require an appropriate work time at each station, and appropriate rest time between stations, to be established. The work to rest ratio will need to be geared towards the target group. Guidelines for appropriate work to rest ratios for different fitness levels are outlined in Chapter 5.

The time-controlled circuit using a stopwatch

One method of timing the work and rest time is to use a stopwatch. An advantage of this approach is that it allows for the same work time to be spent at each station, and the same rest time to be maintained between each station. A disadvantage is that more attention may be paid to watching the clock rather than observing participants. However, when the teacher becomes more proficient, it is often possible for them to estimate the time, rather than clock-watch.

The time-controlled circuit using an exercise station

An alternative method of controlling the circuit is by using a specific exercise station to dictate the time. For example, if shuttle runs are used as a station, a set number of runs can be performed before moving on to the next station. An advantage of this approach is that it gives the teacher more freedom to observe and correct. A key disadvantage of using this approach is that different participants will perform the activity at different speeds. If some participants take longer, then the overall work time on each station will vary slightly.

The time-controlled circuit using a pre-recorded tape

Another method of managing the work time is to use a pre-recorded tape. These can be purchased from the numerous companies that record music tapes for the fitness industry (addresses are listed at the back of this book). One advantage of using these tapes is that the work time at each station and rest time between stations can be controlled by the playing time and breaks in the music. Another advantage is that the timing of work and rest ratios at each station will be the same. In addition, it gives the teacher freedom to observe and correct. A disadvantage is that, as the class participants progress, the work time cannot be increased as the tapes are pre-recorded. Therefore, to achieve progression, one needs to either purchase a tape with a longer work period or increase the intensity of the exercise stations themselves.

The time-controlled circuit using a lighting system

Another method of managing the work to rest ratio of a circuit is to use a lighting system (similar to traffic lights). When the light comes on, work starts on the station, and when the lights go out, participants change stations.

The time-controlled circuit split group control

Another variation of a time-controlled circuit is to split the group. Half the group perform the circuit stations and the other half perform a timed control exercise. This method requires the group to work in pairs, with one partner performing the circuit station and the other performing an exercise dictated by the teacher. The partners swap positions once the control exercise has been performed. This type of circuit works very well if the stations are of a muscular strength and endurance bias, and the control exercises are of a cardiovascular bias. It ensures all components of fitness are trained and that intensity is sufficiently maintained.

Summary of the advantages and disadvantages of using a timed approach to controlling the circuit

A benefit of fixing the time spent on exercise stations is that all participants move on to the next station at the same time. There are no queues between stations. A disadvantage is that participants may try to compete with each other to perform more repetitions. This may lead to exercise stations being executed poorly.

Participants should therefore be encouraged to perform at a comfortable pace and through a full range of motion. It should be noted that a competition circuit utilises competition as a method of progressing the circuit for fitter participants. This approach is explained on page 42.

The repetition-controlled circuit

There are two main approaches of controlling the repetitions performed. Either the teacher can dictate a set repetition range (e.g. 20 repetitions of each exercise) or they can allow participants to select from between two and four different repetition ranges (e.g. choose to perform either 8, 12, 16 or 20 repetitions of each exercise).

If the teacher sets only one number of repetitions, the number they suggest may not be appropriate for different abilities. However, this need not be a problem. Different intensities can be offered, and participants can be advised to select an appropriate intensity for the prescribed repetitions. People may perform at different speeds, however, and some may finish the exercise before others. They will therefore be inactive while they wait for others to finish, and queues may develop at specific stations. This is equally a problem if a selection of repetition ranges is offered.

The best way to avoid the occurrence of queues is to have a control exercise in the middle of the room. Participants should perform the control exercise while they wait for the rest of the group to complete their exercise. When the whole group are in the middle of the room, everyone can move on to the next station.

Summary of methods of controlling work time at each station

- Stopwatch-timed
- Exercise station-timed
- Music tape-timed
- Lighting system-timed
- Split group-timed
- Exercise repetition prescribed by teacher
- Exercise repetition-timed, selected by participants

Layout and arrangement of circuit stations

There are numerous ways of shaping the circuit. The format selected should accommodate the number of participants and cater for their different abilities. If dealing with smaller groups or beginners it is unwise to have a large number of stations with only one person exercising on each. This makes it difficult for the teacher to manage and to move around, observe and correct, and it is also not conducive to developing a collaborative workout atmosphere. It is therefore advisable to encourage smaller groups of people to perform at each station to assist with group motivation, and observation. A variety of circuit formats/shapes are illustrated in Figures 4.1 to 4.9. The advantages and disadvantages of each of these formats are identified. Note: X indicates the position of class participants.

Fig 4.1 Traditional square/rectangular-shaped circuit format

1	2	3	4
xxxx	xxxx	xxxx	xxxx
xxxx	xxxx	xxxx	xxxx
5	6	7	8

Fig 4.2 Lined circuit

1	2	3	4	5	6	7	8
×	×	×	×	×	×	×	×
×	×	×	×	×	×	×	×
×	×	×	×	×	×	×	×
×	×	×	×	×	×	×	×
×	×	×	×	×	×	×	×
×	×	×	×	×	×	×	×
×	×	×	×	×	×	×	×

NB: this is an example of an eight-station muscular strength and endurance-biased circuit. To challenge cardiovascular fitness use the exercises illustrated in Chapter 9.

NB: this is an example of an eight-station cardiovascular circuit using little equipment (only steps). If no equipment is available another exercise from those illustrated in Chapter 9 can be used.

To work muscular strength and endurance, use the exercises illustrated at the end of Chapter 11.

Advantages

- Enables a large number and variety of exercise stations
- Variety of stations will maintain interest and assist motivation
- Can be very challenging, so ideal for fitter participants
- A variety of equipment can be used
- Can be used for cardiovascular- and muscular strength and endurance-biased sessions provided exercises are planned effectively, i.e. alternating and spacing stations so that intensity is maintained.

Disadvantages

- More difficult for the teacher to move around and observe if a large number of stations are used
- Difficult to instruct and coach beginners unless all are placed on the same station. This may draw the teacher's attention away from the rest of the class and embarrass those people who are the centre of the teacher's attention.

Advantages

- Ideal for cardiovascular circuits
- Relatively easy for the teacher to move around and observe.

Disadvantages

- Difficult, if not impossible, to organise and use equipment for this approach
- Not as effective for muscular strength and endurance training, but not impossible or inappropriate.

Fig 4.3 Corners circuit	
1	2
XXXX	XXXX
XXXX	XXXX
XXXX	XXXX
XXXX	XXXX
XXXX	XXXX
XXXX	XXXX
3	4

Fig 4.4 Half split circuit	
1	2
XXXXXXXXX	XXXXXXXXX
XXXXXXXXX	XXXXXXXXX
XXXXXXXXX	XXXXXXXXX
XXXXXXXXX	XXXXXXXXX
XXXXXXXXX	XXXXXXXXX
XXXXXXXXX	XXXXXXXXX
XXXXXXXXX	XXXXXXXXX
XXXXXXXXX	XXXXXXXXX

NB: this is an example of an eight-station combined muscular strength and endurance and cardiovascular circuit. Participants need to move around the circuit at least twice to ensure all exercise stations are performed.

Exercise stations can be reduced in number, time, etc. for beginners.

Advantages

- Works well for cardiovascular circuits.
- Easier to manage because fewer stations.
- Ideal for smaller groups.
- Suitable for beginners – fewer exercises to remember and repetition could improve performance.
- Very small groups can perform at one station and the coach can move around with them to assist performance.

Disadvantages

- May become too repetitious or boring if the same stations are repeated for a number of circuits.

NB: the teacher instructs one half of the group to perform one exercise (e.g. press-ups) while the other half of the group performs another exercise (e.g. knee lifts). The exercises selected should be planned in advance and either a list placed on the wall or the teacher and class work from memory.

Advantages

- Ideal for cardiovascular circuits
- Can work well if one half of the group perform cardiovascular exercise and the other half perform muscular strength and endurance exercise
- Easier to manage – only two exercises being performed at the same time
- Easy to lead and instruct as fewer exercises to explain
- Ideal for beginners
- Potentially easier to observe and correct
- Can vary exercises to maintain desired training effect
- Only instructions/commands and coaching points for two exercises need to be given.

Disadvantages:

- May need a spotter to observe one half of the group if complex exercises are used

- Need to vary the exercises to create interest, prevent boredom and ensure a balanced workout is achieved.

Fig 4.5 Command-led circuit

NB: in a command-led circuit the teacher instructs the participants which exercise to do from a list of exercises displayed on the wall or from memory. The exercises would be planned in advance.

Advantages

- All participants perform the same activity at the same time so potentially easier to manage
- More appropriate for beginners, since all participants are performing the same exercise.
- Easier to observe and correct
- Can vary exercises and maintain desired training effect
- Only instructions/commands and coaching points for one exercise need to be given at any one time
- No circuit cards are needed – participants follow teacher's commands and demonstrations
- An effective way of introducing circuit stations as part of a refresher session
- Allows flexibility. The teacher can change exercises to suit the needs of the group and offer alternatives for different abilities in the same session. They can also start or finish the exercises at a timed interval to accommodate the requirements of the group
- Easy to train all components of fitness.

Participants can be instructed to perform a muscular strength and endurance exercise between cardiovascular exercises
- Easier to control large groups.

Disadvantages

- Can be regimental. The teacher may appear to be dictating instructions
- Can only use equipment if there is sufficient available for every participant
- Can be strenuous and may be inappropriate for less fit individuals. This will depend on the exercises planned, how they are instructed, whether alternatives are offered and, of course, the sensitivity and awareness of the teacher.

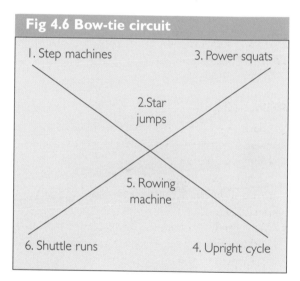

Fig 4.6 Bow-tie circuit

1. Step machines
3. Power squats
2. Star jumps
5. Rowing machine
6. Shuttle runs
4. Upright cycle

NB: this is an example of a six-station cardiovascular circuit using cardiovascular machines and other equipment. If such equipment is not available, the cardiovascular exercises illustrated in Chapter 9 can be used to replace machine exercises. For a muscular strength and endurance-biased circuit, use the exercises illustrated in Chapter 11.

Advantages

- Can get quite a few exercises in a small space
- If CV kit is used, a superset approach can be used for other stations:

CV machines	Station 2	Station 3
	Star jumps	Ab curl
	Lunges	Back extension
	Calf raises	Reverse curl
5 mins	Squats	Tricep dip
	Back lunges	Press-up
	1 min each	1 min each

Disadvantages

- Can be confusing, harder to lead or manage
- Participants need careful direction re: order of stations.

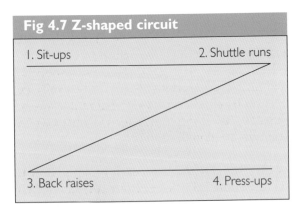

Fig 4.7 Z-shaped circuit

1. Sit-ups   2. Shuttle runs

3. Back raises   4. Press-ups

Advantages

- Easy to manage/lead
- Can get a lot of participants into a fairly small space, so easier to observe.

Disadvantages

- Need to allow enough space between stations to avoid overcrowding, which makes it harder to observe
- Takes time to set up if equipment is used
- Participants need to have the order of the stations carefully explained.

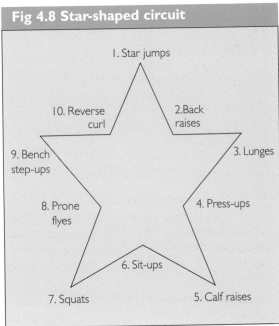

Fig 4.8 Star-shaped circuit

1. Star jumps
2. Back raises
3. Lunges
4. Press-ups
5. Calf raises
6. Sit-ups
7. Squats
8. Prone flyes
9. Bench step-ups
10. Reverse curl

Advantages

- Utilises space well
- All CV exercises/leg exercises are on the outside
- All MSE exercises are on the inside
- A lot of people can be fitted into a small area.

Disadvantages

- Need to allow space for equipment/mats etc.
- Need to plan exercises carefully
- Participants need careful direction to order of stations.

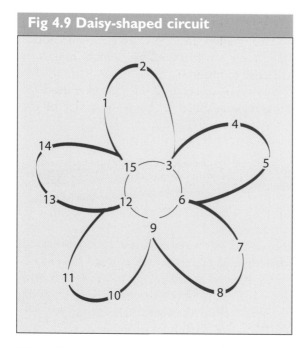

Fig 4.9 Daisy-shaped circuit

NB: 10-station outside circuit with muscular and strength endurance bias – 30–45 secs work time on each station; five-station inside circuit with aerobic bias: 60–90 secs work time on each station.

Perform two muscular strength and endurance exercises, then move to centre to perform an aerobic exercise, then move on to the next two muscular strength and endurance stations, etc.

Progressive approaches to circuit training

Once participants have achieved an appropriate level of competence and fitness the circuit will need to be progressed and varied to maintain interest and maintain and develop fitness and skill. Methods of progressing the circuit are discussed below.

Work, rest and play circuit

For a work, rest and play circuit the participants need to be organised into small sub-groups with three people in each group:

- Participant one performs the work station which is a muscular strength and endurance-bias exercise
- Participant two rests and motivates the other two participants in his/her sub-group while jogging on the spot or skipping
- Participant three performs the play station, which is an aerobic-bias exercise.

An alternative way of organising this type of circuit is to split the whole group into three large groups. The first group perform the muscular strength and endurance activity. The second group perform an aerobic activity. The third group jog around the circuit area.

This type of circuit is best managed using a timed approach. For example, performing each of the three phases (work, then rest, then play) for 45 secs. Once each phase has been completed by all sub-group members, the exercise stations can be changed or the sub-group can move on to the next group of stations. As a guideline, there can generally be approximately five to eight different exercise changes. An example of exercises that can be used are listed in Table 4.1.

In the example provided, each group performs each station (all three exercises) and then moves on to the next station. This continues until all exercises have been completed.

Obstacle circuit

In this circuit design an obstacle is completed before/between each exercise. The obstacle is designed to work the same or a similar muscle

Table 4.1	Example of a work, rest and play circuit		
Station	**Work**	**Rest**	**Play**
Station 1	Press-ups	Run around circuit	Jumping jumps
Station 2	Sit-ups	Jog and motivate	Spotty dogs
Station 3	Back raises	Run around circuit	Knee lifts
Station 4	Squats	Jog and motivate	Leg kicks
Station 5	Prone flyes	Run around circuit	Forward lunges

group as the next exercise, the aim being to pre-exhaust the muscle group with the obstacle before working that muscle again on the specific work station. For example, mats and benches or steps are used to create a tunnel which participants crawl through. Having crawled through the tunnel on their tummies using their arms to pull them through, they then move on to the work station. The station, e.g. a seated row using rubber bands, is marked for a certain number of repetitions. Participants then move back through the tunnel. The obstacle and work station are continued for a certain amount of time (one to two minutes). Participants then move on to the next obstacle and work station.

NB: pre-exhausting a specific muscle group before working that muscle group again is an advanced method of training. It should only be used with participants who have a good level of fitness and those who are able to maintain correct exercise technique throughout.

Overtaking circuit

In an overtaking circuit participants start off at different intervals or stations around the circuit. The aim of this circuit is for each participant to try to overtake the person in front having completed the same amount of repetitions or work time as the person(s) they are chasing.

An obvious disadvantage of this approach is that participants may focus more on performing at speed rather than on their technique. The teacher must therefore observe carefully and provide sufficient coaching reinforcement.

NB: it is also essential that this approach is only implemented once participants are able to perform all the exercises with safe and effective exercise technique. This is not an appropriate approach to be used with beginners to circuit training.

Competition circuit

To organise a competition circuit, participants need to be paired off with a partner of similar ability to themselves. The partners move around the circuit competing against each other, the aim being to beat the other's score at each exercise station. The repetitions performed at each station by each participant can also be recorded. This enables participants to compete with themselves as well as their partner at the next visit, and has the advantage of allowing them to monitor their own individual progression carefully.

This type of circuit works most effectively if a time limit is applied to each station. Timed approaches to circuit training are described on pages 34–5.

Colour circuit

The colour circuit is really an alternative method for prescribing repetitions. Each participant follows a specific colour theme through the circuit, based on their current fitness level. There can be as many colours as there are different fitness abilities.
For example:

- green – easy/beginners
- blue – moderate/intermediate
- red – hard/advanced.

Giant sets circuit

A giant sets circuit is best performed using the four sides of a sports hall/studio (see Figure 4.3). Four body parts/muscle groups are selected and three or four exercises are designed to work each. Participants stay at one station and perform each different exercise simultaneously, before moving on to the next body part.

An example of a circuit plan for a super sets circuit would be as follows:

> Station one (abdominals)
> Exercise 1: curl-ups
> Exercise 2: curl-up and twist
> Exercise 3: reverse curls
> Exercise 4: abdominal crunches
>
> Station two: (legs)
> Exercise 1: dead-lift
> Exercise 2: alternate leg lunges
> Exercise 3: step-ups
> Exercise 4: calf raises

> Station three: include exercises to work . . . the chest, shoulders and triceps
>
> Station four: include exercises to work . . . the back and biceps

This design ensures a whole body approach is achieved throughout the workout.

Super sets circuit

Super sets circuit training can be achieved using a similar structure to giant set training but working opposing muscle groups (rather than the same muscle group) at each station. For example:

> Station one
> Exercises for abdominals and erector spinae
>
> Station two
> Exercises for triceps and biceps
>
> Station three
> Exercises for pectorals and trapezius and latisimus dorsi
>
> Station four
> Exercises for quads and hamstrings

Stage training or sets circuit

A more advanced form of circuit training is the 'sets circuit', which is often referred to as 'stage training'. Stage training is a modified, progressive form of circuit training and is the intermediate stage between circuit training and weight training. Rather than visit an exercise station for a set time or number of repetitions and then move on to the next station, the same station is visited several times (2–4 sets) before moving on to the next station.

This allows specific muscle loading which helps develop the training effect on the muscles still further. Prior to starting this type of circuit the exercisers will have to find their training 'requirement'. This is done by performing each exercise within the circuit to ascertain the maximum number of repetitions achievable at any given station or in a given time frame (30–60 secs). Take no more than one minute's rest between each exercise. Once all exercises have been completed, training repetitions can be set. To do this, take the total number of repetitions achieved and halve it: this will be the training requirement for each set. This type of training can be varied by including a super set (agonist followed by antagonist), which will take out any rest interval as the opposing muscle is worked during what would have been the rest interval.

Individual circuit

This circuit is again a variation on a theme, but can be made specific to the individual. It is an opportunity to pit exerciser against the clock while encouraging him/her to maintain good technique.

There are three phases to this type of circuit: the teaching, the testing, and the timing.

Teaching

Using the correct technique, all exercise stations are taught to each individual. They then perform the circuit two to three times round in slow time so that technique can be reinforced.

Testing

Each individual must now be tested in order to set their individual training repetitions. This is achieved by performing each exercise in circuit order to the individual's maximum (allowing no more than one minute's rest between exercises). Exercise selection/intensity should be such that individuals manage to achieve their training overload within that period. When testing is over, maximum repetitions achieved should be recorded alongside each exercise. This number is then halved to arrive at the training repetition prescription, which again is recorded.

NB: it is recommended that training repetitions should be no fewer than six and no more than 25.

Timing

Having had a couple of practice runs around the circuit, first getting used to the exercises and secondly finding a suitable repetition range, the exercisers then need to complete three laps (circuits) at full speed while maintaining good technique. This time is then recorded as the initial time. A realistic 'target' time now needs to be agreed on and recorded. The circuit is then performed regularly until the target time has been achieved. Having achieved this target, retesting must be carried out on the same or a harder circuit and a new 'target' established.

Summary of progressive approaches to circuit training

- Work, rest and play
- Obstacle
- Overtaking
- Competition
- Colour
- Giant sets
- Super sets
- Stage training or sets circuit
- Individual

Summary

Ultimately there are many different approaches that can be adopted to design and lead a circuit training session. This chapter has outlined only some of these approaches. In Part Four, guidelines for designing circuit training sessions for general populations, specific sports, older adults and outdoor circuits are provided.

With a creative mind and a little imagination, many variations on the basic circuit training themes can be designed.

STRUCTURE AND PROGRESSION FOR A CIRCUIT TRAINING SESSION

5

How to structure a circuit training programme

As with all programmes it is essential that the circuit training session is structured correctly. All group training activities should be preceded by an appropriate warm-up and concluded with an appropriate cool-down (see Chapter 6). The main workout should comprise a range of exercises (see Chapters 8 and 10) designed using an appropriate format/arrangement of circuit stations (see Chapter 4) and should accommodate the specific needs and requirements of the group and individuals being taught (see Part Four). An outline of the necessary session structure is provided in Table 5.1.

Considerations necessary when structuring sessions for general populations

For most populations a programme format that targets all the components of physical fitness will be most appropriate. Training all the components provides a more holistic approach to fitness and should therefore meet all the participants' requirements and satisfy most personal fitness goals. A range of exercises appropriate for a complete circuit training programme are illustrated and explained in Part Three with a needs analysis and lesson plans provided in Part Four.

However, the programme will sometimes need to be adapted to suit the special requirements, needs and wants of a particular group (Part Four). If a group of people wishes to train purely to improve cardiovascular fitness, all the exercises illustrated in Chapter 9 will be appropriate for use in the main circuit. Alternatively, if the group wishes to improve muscular strength and endurance, the exercises illustrated in Chapter 11 will be appropriate. If a combined cardiovascular fitness and muscular strength and endurance workout is required, then the exercises in both of the aforementioned chapters are appropriate.

When using a combined approach, it is wise to alternate muscular strength and endurance exercises with cardiovascular exercises. This ensures that the intensity of activity is maintained for an appropriate time to make cardiovascular fitness improvements. This approach is advisable because many of the muscular strength and endurance activities illustrated will not be suitable to maintain the intensity necessary for sufficient cardiovascular training. The intensity may be too low if such exercises are performed consecutively in the same circuit.

An alternative approach is to perform two specific circuits, the first consisting of cardiovascular exercises and the second consisting of muscular strength and endurance exercises. If two main circuits are used, the intensity of the cardiovascular circuit will need to be reduced slightly before going on to the muscular strength and endurance circuit.

Considerations necessary when structuring sessions for special populations

Specialist groups such as older adults and sportspeople will have different needs from the general population. The basic structure of the circuit programme should follow that given in Table 5.1. However, in order to meet the

Table 5.1	The structure of a circuit training session
Warm-up	Mobility and pulse-raising activities Preparatory stretches Re-warming/specific warm-up (increasing intensity to the level of the circuit and introducing the activities to be used throughout the main workout)
Main workout – circuit training component (three approaches)	Specific exercises targeting all major muscle groups to achieve a balanced whole-body approach and improve just muscular strength and endurance; or a range of specific exercises targeted to improve just cardiovascular fitness A combination of exercises to improve both muscular and cardiovascular components of fitness A combination of exercises to improve muscular and cardiovascular fitness and rehearse specific movements for a selected sport
Cool-down	Warming-down exercises (lowering intensity from the level of the circuit). NB: if the nature of the exercises used in the circuit have a cooling effect on the body, it may be necessary to re-warm the muscles at this stage, prior to stretching Post-workout stretches (developmental and maintenance) Relaxation activities (optional) Remobilise

NB: the type and intensity of exercises included in the re-warmer and warm-down will need to correspond to the intensity and purpose of the main workout. If the intensity of the main workout is high and includes a number of energetic cardiovascular movements, then the intensity of these components will need to be built up to and built down from this higher level of intensity.

specific needs of the group it may be necessary to perform a more detailed needs analysis.

A detailed analysis of the needs of three fitness levels – general fitness, older adults and sport-specific – is provided in Part Four. In addition, appropriate exercises and lesson plans for these groups are outlined and illustrated.

How can a circuit training session be adapted for different fitness levels?

The intensity of the individual stations can be adapted to suit different requirements by varying:

- rate – speed of the exercise
- range of motion
- repetitions
- resistance (using longer levers, adding weights, etc.)

- rest – the rest time between each station/ intensity of activity used during the rest period.

NB: detailed progressions are provided for each of the specific exercises illustrated in Part Three.

The intensity of the whole circuit training programme can be adapted to accommodate different needs by varying:

- number of stations
- intensity of the exercises at each station
- time working at each station
- number of times the circuit is performed
- rest time between each circuit.

The timing and intensity of each component will need to be adapted slightly for different groups. Tables 5.2 and 5.3 provide an outline of some of the necessary alterations to session structure, timing and intensity for three general fitness populations.

Table 5.2	An outline of the structure, duration and intensity of components for three general fitness populations		
	Less fit and specialist groups	Intermediate fitness level and general groups	Advanced fitness level and sport-specific groups
Overall duration	45 mins	45–60 mins	60–90 mins
Overall intensity of session components	Low	Moderate	Higher
Speed of movements	Relatively slow pace	Moderate pace	Relatively quick pace
Warm-up component (mobility, pulse-raising, preparatory).	Comparatively lower intensity and longer duration	Moderate intensity and duration	Comparatively high intensity and generally shorter duration
Warm-up exercises	15–20 mins	10–15 mins	10–15 mins

Table 5.2	An outline of the structure, duration and intensity of components for three general fitness populations cont.		
Warm-up exercises cont.	Smaller range of motion for mobility and pulse-raising exercises, building more gradually; slower movements; slower directional changes; simpler movements; easier and more supportive stretch positions (providing balance where possible)	Moderate range of motion, combining some mobility and pulse-raising together; moderate pace and directional moves; some stretch positions may need to be supported; slightly larger range of motion	Combine mobility and pulse-raising; build intensity and skill level much more quickly; movements can be quicker with more directional changes; stretch positions can be more challenging; more pulse-raising between stretches to keep warm and maintain intensity
Main circuit – cardiovascular and MSE exercise stations	15–20 mins Comparatively shorter duration and lower intensity	20–35 mins Moderate duration and moderate intensity	40 mins Longer duration and higher intensity
Exercise stations	See Table 5.3	See Table 5.3	See Table 5.3
Cool-down component (pulse-lowering developmental and maintenance post-workout stretches, relaxation and remobilisation)	10–15 mins Comparatively longer duration and lower intensity	5–10 mins Moderation duration and intensity	5–10 mins Shorter duration and relatively higher intensity
Cool-down and specific exercises	Longer and more gradual pulse-lowering; easier and more supportive stretch positions; shorter held developmental stretches	Moderate timing for pulse-lower; slightly larger range of motion in stretch positions; increase time of hold for developmental stretches; more challenging stretch positions	Intensity of pulse-lower can decrease more rapidly; can combine some maintenance stretch positions; developmental stretches held longer

NB: these timings are only suggested as guidelines and are variable depending on the environment, the requirements of the individual/group and the structural design of the main workout.

Table 5.3	Adapting the intensity and duration of the circuit for different fitness levels		
	Less fit and specialist groups	**Intermediate fitness level and general groups**	**Advanced fitness level and sport-specific groups**
Overall duration of circuit (including warm-up and warm-down	45 mins	45–60 mins	60–90 mins
Overall intensity of circuit session	Low	Moderate–high	High
Work time on stations (NB: if muscular strength is a goal, the time will need to be shorter and the intensity higher)	Shorter	Moderate	Longer
Rest time between stations (NB: cardiovascular circuits will need an active rest. Performing a lower intensity activity between stations should be sufficient	Longer rest time – performing lower intensity activity to allow sufficient recovery	Moderate rests – performing a moderately intense activity to allow recovery from higher intensity activities	Shorter rest time needed between more intense activities. Rest periods can be more active – aim for continuous movement around circuit
Approach (NB: this may vary to accommodate the fitness goals of the individual/group being trained)	Timed or reps. Command format is easier to manage	Timed or reps	Timed or reps to tailor programme to meet specific needs. Some of the more progressive approaches described in Chapters 4 and 5 can be used to add variety and maintain the interest of fitter participants

Table 5.3	Adapting the intensity and duration of the circuit for different fitness levels cont.		
Number of stations (NB: this may vary depending on the number of participants)	Low (4–8)	Moderate (8–12)	Higher (10–20 or more, depending on aims of circuit, number of participants and available space)
Number of circuits (NB: this will vary depending on the number of stations)	Low (1–2)	Moderate (1–3)	Higher (1–4)
Appropriate exercises (see Part Four for how to perform these)	Compound (working a number of muscles to reduce the number of exercises); simpler exercises with less impact/resistance	Compound and isolated exercises using equipment; adding more complexity, some impact and greater resistance	Compound and isolation exercises using equipment; more complex activities with higher impact/ resistance

STRUCTURE OF A CIRCUIT TRAINING SESSION WITH CIRCUIT TRAINING EXERCISES

PART THREE

INTRODUCTION

This section of the book discusses the appropriate structure for a circuit training session. It explains the purpose of warming up and cooling down with illustrations of appropriate exercises for mobility, pulse raising (or lowering) and stretching. It also explains the aims of cardiovascular and muscular strength and endurance training as part of the main circuit session with illustrations of a range of exercises that can be included to train these components of fitness both with and without equipment (e.g. steps and stability balls).

The exercises used and structure of the circuit should reflect the goals and needs of participants. They should also improve the intended components of fitness (introduced in Part One).

It should be noted that there are many other possible exercises and variations to all the exercises listed. It is hoped that sufficient are given to provide an effective resource for teachers to plan their programmes for a number of months.

NB: Key teaching and postural points are explained throughout. As a general guideline, see box for postural advice that applies to most exercises.

Each exercise description provides:

- an illustration of the exercise
- the purpose/benefit of performing the exercise
- the starting position and key instructions

Correct postural alignment

- Pelvis neutral – keeping pelvic bones and pubic bones level (no forward or backward tilt).
- Abdominal muscles engaged to maintain a fixed position of the lower spine.
- The spine should be kept lengthened and upright.
- The shoulders should be relaxed and down, keeping a space between the shoulders and ears.
- The chest should be lifted without pushing the rib cage forwards.
- The head should be up, with eyes looking forward and chin parallel to the floor.
- The knees should be unlocked.
- Breathing should be comfortable throughout all exercises. For muscular strength and endurance exercises, breathe out on the effort (lifting or concentric) phase of the exercise.

- the essential coaching points for ensuring the exercise is performed safely and effectively
- a range of progressions and adaptations to add variety and make the exercises suitable for different abilities, needs and populations.

Other points to note:

- Some pulse-raising exercises used in the warm-up can be adapted and made more intense so that they can be used within the circuit to improve cardiovascular fitness (Chapter 6). This is outlined where possible.
- Additional arm lines can be used with

cardiovascular movements to add variety to the movements; these are outlined at the end of Chapter 9.

- Each of the muscular strength and endurance arm movements (shoulder press, chest press) can be used as an arm line without the use of weights. This is useful for skill rehearsal in the warm up (re-warming phase).
- Further variation to muscular strength and endurance exercises can be achieved by altering the speed. For example, two counts up and two counts down (or four counts up and four counts down). This requires the muscles to contract for longer, so it is more controlled and also harder. Alternatively, place more emphasis on the negative (eccentric) phase – three or seven counts down and one count up or the reverse to work on the positive (concentric) phase – three or seven counts up and one down.

WARMING UP AND COOLING DOWN

6

This chapter outlines the effects of warming up and cooling down on the body. It also outlines how to structure these components safely and effectively and illustrates appropriate exercises that can be used for warming up and cooling down.

- enhance our performance
- reduce the risk of injury
- improve the effectiveness of the main workout through adequate preparation

Why do we need to warm up before the main workout?

We need to warm up prior to activity in order to prepare the body's systems for the activities that will follow. Warming up will potentially:

What type of exercises should the warm-up contain?

The warm-up needs to prepare the joints, muscles, heart, circulatory and neuromuscular systems for the main workout. It should therefore contain exercises that achieve the desired effects, outlined in the box below, and

An outline of the desired effects of the warm-up on the body

The warm-up should contain exercises that:
- promote the release of synovial fluid into the joint capsule and warm the tendons, muscles and ligaments which surround each joint. This will ensure the joints are adequately lubricated and cushioned, and will allow a fuller range of motion to be achieved at each joint. This can be achieved by mobility exercises
- increase the heart rate, promote an increase of blood flow to the muscles and an increase in the delivery of oxygen. This will make the body warmer and the muscles more pliable, and will allow them to work more comfortably throughout the main workout. This can be achieved by pulse-raising exercises
- lengthen the muscles and move them through a larger range of motion. This will allow them to contract more effectively in the main workout and may lower the risk of injury if moving into extended positions in the main workout. This can be achieved by stretching exercises
- activate the brain and neuromuscular pathways, focusing attention and concentration, rehearsing skills and movement patterns, rehearsing the muscle and joint actions in the way they are to be moved in the main workout, and raising the heart rate to a desired training level. This can be achieved by re-warming exercises

Table 6.1	Actions possible at each joint area and appropriate warm-up exercises to achieve each action	
Joint area	**Joint actions possible**	**Appropriate exercises**
Ankle	Plantar flexion and dorsiflexion	Heel and toe alternately pointing to the floor – exercise 6.7 (page 67)
		Walking/pedalling through the feet – exercise 6.11 (page 71)
		Rotating/circling the foot
Knee	Flexion and extension	Squats – exercise 6.9 (page 69)
		Leg curls – exercise 6.5 (page 65)
Hip	Flexion and extension	Lifting the knees up towards the chest and down again – exercise 6.6 (page 66)
		Back lunges – exercise 9.19 (page 113)
	Abduction and adduction	Taking the leg out to the side and back in (low-impact jumping jacks) – exercise 9.1 (page 95)
	Rotation	Standing upright, raising one foot slightly off the ground and rotating that leg inwards and outwards under control
Spine	Lateral flexion and extension	Side bends – 6.2 (page 62)
	Rotation	Side twists – 6.3 (page 63)
	Flexion and extension	Humping and hollowing the spine – exercise 6.4 (page 64)

Table 6.1	Actions possible at each joint area and appropriate warm-up exercises to achieve each action cont.	
Shoulder and shoulder girdle	Elevation and depression	Lifting and lowering the shoulders – exercise 6.1 (page 61)
	Abduction and adduction	Taking the arms out to the side of the body and back in – exercise 9.22 (page 115)
	Rotation	Rotating the arm in a figure-of-eight motion towards and away from the body (with or without weights)
	Horizontal flexion and extension	Pec decs' – exercise 9.26 (page 115)
	Circumduction	Moving the arm in a complete circle
Elbow	Flexion, extension and rotation	Bending and straightening the elbow – exercises 6.3 (page 63)

reflect the activities that are to be used in the main workout.

How should the warm-up be structured for a circuit training session?

The warm-up should be structured in three stages:

1. Mobility and pulse-raising exercises (a general warm-up) – see Table 6.1 and exercises listed at the end of this chapter (pages 68–71)

2. Short stretches – see exercises listed at the end of chapter

3. Re-warmer (a specific warm-up for the circuit to be performed with an introduction to the circuit stations to be performed) – see pulse-raising exercises on pages 68–71), which can be performed at a slightly higher intensity, and Chapters 9 and 11 for cardiovascular and muscular strength and endurance activities to be performed in the main workout at a slightly lower intensity. The intensity can build progressively.

Summary of the guidelines for planning the warm-up

- Start with smaller mobility and pulse-raising exercises and gradually build up the range of motion and intensity of the movements. This can be achieved by progressively moving through a larger range of motion, bending deeper, travelling more and moving at a progressively faster pace
- Combine static mobility exercises with larger pulse-raising movements for groups with greater skill, to create interest and maintain the pace of the warm-up
- Mobilise all joints to be used in the main workout
- Use lower impact, pulse-raising moves since these are less stressful for the body
- Ensure that the body is fully warm before stretching and moving to a larger range of motion
- Ensure all the muscles to be used in the main workout are stretched
- Combine static stretches with larger pulse-raising movements to maintain the pace of the warm-up and prevent the body from cooling down
- Allow time for the learning and rehearsal of skills related to activities that will be part of the main circuit. The teacher should introduce and demonstrate more complex exercises and allow rehearsal
- Ensure the intensity of the re-warm builds gradually to the level of the main circuit.

What type of exercises should the cool-down contain?

The cool-down should contain exercises that:
- gradually return and lower the heart rate to a pre-exercise level. This reduces the stress on the heart muscle. It also promotes the return of venous blood to the heart and lowers the risk of blood pooling. This can be achieved by pulse-lowering/cooling down exercises. The pulse-raising exercises illustrated in Part Four are appropriate if they are performed at a higher level initially and gradually reduced in size and speed
- return the muscles back to their normal state. This will maintain the flexibility and range of motion of the muscles and joints. This can be achieved by static maintenance stretches (held for approximately 10–15 secs)
- increase the length of the muscles. This will increase the flexibility and range of motion of the joints and muscles. This can be achieved by static developmental stretches. To develop the stretch, take the muscle to the point of feeling mild tension and when the tension eases extend further into the stretch and hold for a longer period of time (15 secs-plus)
- relax the body and mind. This will help to reduce stress and promote a feeling of calm. This can be achieved by specific relaxation techniques, such as tensing and releasing the muscles, allowing the body to rest and be still and focusing on the breathing. Techniques for relaxation are explained in the *Complete Guide to Exercising Away Stress*, Lawrence (A&C Black: 2005)
- revitalise the body and mind. This will leave the body feeling rejuvenated and ready to return to normal activities. This can be achieved by gentle remobilizing exercises. Gentle mobility and pulse-raising exercises will bring about the desired result.

Summary of the guidelines for planning the cool-down

- Start with higher intensity exercises and gradually bring down the range of motion and intensity of the movements. This can be achieved by progressively decreasing the amount of jumping, bending and travelling movements, and moving at a progressively slower pace. If the main workout consists of mostly muscular strength and endurance exercises, it is possible that the body will have cooled down. Therefore, it may be necessary to actually re-warm the body before stretching, rather than cooling down
- Maintenance stretches should be included for all the muscles worked in the main workout
- Developmental stretches should be included for muscle groups which lack a full range of motion. Comfortable and supportive positions should be used when developing a stretch and the muscle must be sufficiently warm. To develop flexibility, the stretches need to be taken to the point where a mild tension is felt. Once tension eases, move further into position. The muscle should be allowed to relax again and held for between 15–30 secs, depending on comfort
- Only include specific relaxation exercises if the environment is warm. Specific active muscular relaxation techniques, such as tense and release (where muscles are tightened and then relaxed individually), and extend and release (where one body part is extended away from another body part creating a lengthening feeling), are effective
- For remobilising use gentle activities that will enliven the body and mind and finish the session on a positive note.

Why do we need to cool down after the main workout?

Cooling down after the main workout is important to return all the body's systems to their pre-exercise state. Cooling down will:

- lower the heart rate
- reduce body temperature
- prevent muscle soreness
- lengthen muscles
- rejuvenate the mind and body.

How should the cool-down be structured?

The cool-down should be structured in four stages:

1. Cooling down/pulse-lowering exercises (the pulse-raising exercises listed at the end of this chapter can be used, starting at higher intensity and progressively lowering intensity)
2. Post-workout stretches – maintenance and developmental (the stretching exercises listed at the end of this section can be used)
3. Relaxation
4. Remobilise.

Warm-up and cool-down exercises

For a summary of possible joint actions for warm-up exercises, refer back to Table 6.1 on page 57–8.

Exercise 6.1	Shoulder lifts and rolls (mobility)

Purpose

These exercises mobilise the shoulder joint and can be performed with the pulse-raising exercises described for variety if participants have sufficient motor skills.

Starting position and instructions

- Start with the feet hip-width apart
- Shoulder lifts – lift alternate shoulders towards the ears or both shoulders together
- Shoulder rolls – roll alternate shoulders backwards or roll both shoulders together.

These exercises can be performed while walking around or with knee bends. They can also be performed with leg curls or a step and tap movement where the body weight is shifted from one side to the other.

These exercises should be performed for the desired number of repetitions.

Coaching points

- Maintain an upright posture with the back straight and chest lifted
- Keep the hips facing forwards and tighten the abdominal muscles
- Keep the knee joints unlocked
- Move the shoulders at a controlled speed and aim to progress to a larger range of motion.

Progressions/Adaptations

- Start with a small range of motion and progressively increase the range
- Move at a progressively quicker tempo
- Use longer levers by moving the elbow or the full arm around for shoulder rolls
- Vary the speed and/or combine the movements together, e.g., lift the shoulders together, slowly performing two repetitions for eight counts and then alternate shoulder rolls at a quicker pace for eight counts
- Combine the shoulder mobility exercises with other mobility or pulse-raising exercises once skill level increases.

Exercise 6.2	Side bends (mobility)

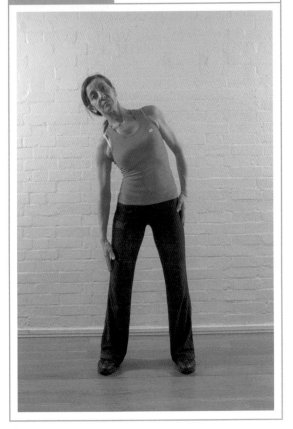

Purpose

This exercise will mobilise the thoracic vertebrae of the spine.

Starting position and instructions

- Start with the feet hip-width apart, the body upright and the knees unlocked
- Bend directly to the right side in a controlled manner
- Return to the central position
- Bend directly to the left side in a controlled manner
- Return to the central position
- Perform the desired number of repetitions.

Coaching points

- Bend only as far over as is comfortable
- Keep the hips facing forwards and avoid hollowing of the lower back by tightening the abdominal muscles
- Keep the movement controlled
- Keep the body lifted between the hips and the ribs
- Lift up before bending to the side
- Lean directly to the side and ensure the body does not roll forwards or backwards
- Visualise your body as being placed between two panes of glass.

Progressions/Adaptations

- Start with a smaller bend and progress to a slightly larger range of motion, but only as far as is comfortable
- Alternate the bending movement from right to left and progress by performing more repetitions to one side before changing side. This will require slightly greater muscular endurance to maintain correct alignment
- Move at a slightly quicker pace. Take care not to move too fast and create excessive momentum as this may cause the movement to become ballistic
- Vary the speed by performing one slow side bend in each direction (down and up to centre, down and up to centre – eight counts total) and then perform four quick, single bends without the pause at the central start position. This will require greater skill from participants
- Perform with knee bends or while walking around when skill level increases.

Exercise 6.3	Side twists (spine mobility)

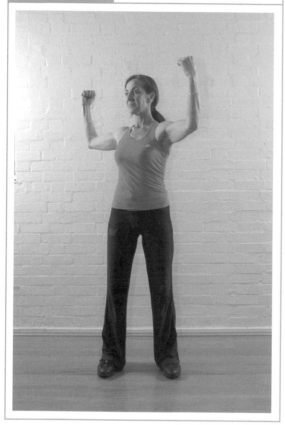

Purpose

This exercise will mobilise the thoracic vertebrae of the spine.

Starting position and instructions

- Start with the feet shoulder-width-and-a-half apart.

- Hold the arms at shoulder level with the elbows slightly bent or place the hands on the hips
- Twist around to one side, back to the centre and then twist to the other side.

Coaching points

- Keep the hips and knees facing forwards, do not let the knee joints roll inwards
- Keep the knees slightly bent
- Make sure the lower back does not twist.
- Keep the abdominals pulled in, the chest lifted, shoulders relaxed and back straight.

Progressions/Adaptations

- Start slow and work through a smaller range of motion. Progressively increase the speed of the movement and move through a slightly larger range of motion. NB: ensure that the speed of movement remains appropriately controlled and that the range of motion is within that range which allows for correct spinal alignment to be maintained
- Keep the hands on the hips instead of held high to take out any fixator work of the deltoid (shoulder) muscles
- Combine the movement with knee bends when skill level increases.

Exercise 6.4	Hump and hollow (spine mobility)

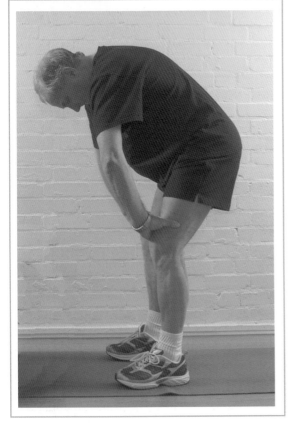

NB: ensure the body is adequately warmed up before moving to this more extended range of motion.

Purpose

This exercise will mobilise the lumbar vertebrae of the spine.

Starting position and instructions

- Start with the feet shoulder-width-and-a-half apart and the knees slightly bent
- Lean the body forwards and place the hands on the knees

- Round the back upwards, contracting the abdominals and humping the spine
- Release under control and return the back to a flattened position.

Coaching points

- Keep the hips and knees facing forwards – do not let the knee joint roll inwards
- Keep the knees slightly bent
- Make sure the lower back does not hollow or twist
- Keep the body weight supported throughout the movement by placing the hands on the thighs
- Keep the abdominals pulled in, the chest lifted and shoulders relaxed.

Progressions/Adaptations

- Start by standing upright, just rounding the shoulders and upper back forwards and backwards
- Progress to placing the hands on the thighs, keeping the back supported and rounding and flattening the spine
- Progressively increase the speed of the movement and move through a slightly larger range of motion. NB: ensure that the speed of movement remains appropriately controlled and that the range of motion is within that range which allows for correct spinal alignment to be maintained
- As a variation, press alternate shoulders forwards, i.e. right shoulder to left knee and left shoulder to right knee, but taking care not to hollow the spine or twist too far and too quickly.

Exercise 6.5	Leg curls (mobility)

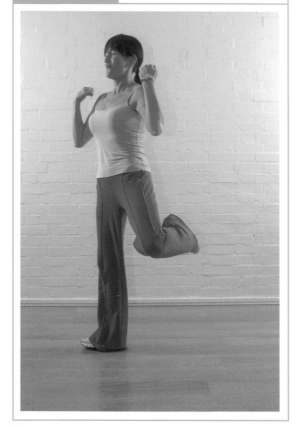

Purpose

This exercise primarily assists with mobilising the knee joints. It will also assist with raising the pulse and warming the muscles since the muscles of the legs will be weight-bearing to transfer the weight of the body from one side to the other.

If it is performed with a greater intensity (travelling or bending deeper) or with impact (jumping) it can effectively be used as a circuit station to improve cardiovascular fitness.

Starting position and instructions

- Start with the feet hip-width apart
- Step out to the right and transfer the weight over to the right leg, kicking the left heel towards the buttocks
- Step the left leg down and transfer the weight over to the left leg, kicking the right heel to the buttocks
- Perform these alternating leg curls for the desired number of repetitions.

Coaching points

- Take a large but comfortable stride of the legs
- Keep the hips facing forwards and avoid hollowing of the lower back by tightening the abdominal muscles
- Ensure the knee joint remains unlocked when landing
- Ensure the knees move in line with the toes and do not roll inwards
- Keep the back straight and the chest lifted
- Keep the movement controlled, smooth and not jerky
- If the exercise is used for cardiovascular training and impact is added, make sure the heels go down to cushion the movement.

Progressions/Adaptations

- Start with a smaller stride and progressively increase stride length but ensure the distance is comfortable and maintains correct alignment
- Move at a progressively quicker pace
- Bend deeper to promote greater pulse-raising
- Travel the movement forwards and backwards; this will add intensity because the body weight is being shifted across gravity. Progress further by travelling a greater distance in each direction
- Perform two or more leg curls to the same side. This requires greater muscular endurance and will require different motor skills
- Add a turn to the movement, e.g. turning the body around to face each different wall in the room on each heel lift: face right as left heel lifts, face back as right heel lifts, face left as left heel lifts, and face front as right heel lifts.

Exercise 6.6	Knee lifts (mobility)

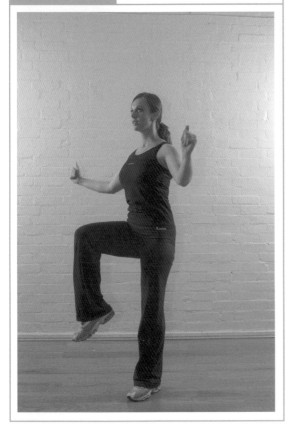

Purpose

This exercise mobilises the hip joints. It will assist with raising the pulse and warming the muscles because the legs are bearing the body weight throughout the movement.

If it is performed with a greater intensity (bending deeper or travelling) or with impact (jumping) it can effectively be used as a circuit station to improve cardiovascular fitness.

Starting position and instructions

- Start with the feet hip-width apart
- Step and shift the weight onto the right leg, lifting the left knee to hip height
- Step and shift the weight onto the left leg, lifting the right knee to hip height
- Perform these alternating knee lifts for the desired number of repetitions.

Coaching points

- Take a comfortable stride of the legs
- Keep the hips facing forwards and avoid hollowing of the lower back by tightening the abdominal muscles
- Keep the knee joints unlocked and ensure the knees stay in line with the toes
- Lift the leg only to a height where an upright spine alignment can be maintained
- Keep the chest lifted and do not allow the body to bend forwards as the leg lifts
- If impact is added, make sure the heels go down to cushion the movement.

Progressions/Adaptations

- Start by lifting the leg only to a small height and progressively lift the leg higher
- Bend the weight-bearing leg a little deeper to add intensity
- Move at a slightly faster pace
- Turn the movement in a circle (as described for leg curls – exercise 6.5 on page 65). This will add variety and challenge motor skills
- Perform two or more repetitions on the same side. This requires greater muscular endurance
- Travel the movement forwards and backwards to achieve a greater pulse-raising effect. Increase this further by travelling a greater distance and increasing the number of repetitions in one direction
- For cardiovascular training, increase intensity by adding impact to shift the resistance of the body upwards against gravity
- To add further intensity for cardiovascular training, perform four or more repetitions on each side and travel the movement in the direction that the knee is lifting.

Exercise 6.7	Heel and toe (mobility)

Purpose

This exercise mobilises the ankle joints. NB: if performed with the weight-bearing leg hopping, that exercise can be used as a cardiovascular exercise.

Starting position and instructions

- Start with the feet hip-width apart and take the weight onto one leg
- Dig the heel of the foot towards the floor and then point the toe towards the floor
- Repeat for the desired number of repetitions and perform on the other leg.

Coaching points

- Keep the weight-bearing leg soft and do not allow the knee to roll in
- Keep the hips facing forwards and the back straight
- Keep the movement controlled
- Keep the knee joints unlocked and ensure the knees move in line with the toes
- Aim for the heel and toe to land in the same place to ensure full range of motion of the ankle is achieved
- If impact is added, make sure the heels go down to cushion the movement.

Progressions/Adaptations

- Start with a smaller range of motion and progress to a larger range of motion
- Move at a progressively faster pace
- Perform fewer repetitions on each side to increase motor skills
- Perform more repetitions on each side to increase muscular endurance

- Add a movement of the upper body to increase motor skills, e.g. a biceps curl
- Circle the ankle as a variation
- Bend and straighten the weight-bearing leg to improve motor skills and to maintain the tempo of the session.

Exercise 6.8	Scoops (pulse-raising)

Purpose

This exercise primarily assists with raising the pulse and warming the muscles. If it is performed with a greater intensity or with impact it can effectively be used to improve cardiovascular fitness.

Starting position and instructions

- Start with the feet hip-width apart
- Step diagonally forwards to the right corner with the right leg leading. Draw the left leg in to meet the right
- Repeat, stepping diagonally forwards to the left side with the left leg leading
- Perform these alternating diagonal scoops for the desired number of repetitions
- The movement can also be performed in reverse.

Coaching points

- Take a large but comfortable stride of the legs
- Keep the hips facing forwards and avoid hollowing of the lower back by tightening the abdominal muscles
- Keep movements of the shoulder joints controlled
- Keep the knee joints unlocked and ensure the knees move in line with the toes
- If impact is added, make sure the heels go down to cushion the movement.

Progressions/Adaptations

- Start with a smaller stride and progressively increase stride length
- Move at a progressively faster pace
- Travel a greater distance by increasing the number of repetitions in one direction

- Perform two or more scoops in the same direction to vary skills
- Increase intensity by adding impact and jumping higher to shift the resistance of the body upwards and against the force of gravity
- Vary the speed, i.e. perform one slow power scoop right (two counts) and one slow power scoop left (two counts), then perform four quick, single count scoops
- Travel the movement forwards or backwards for a set number of counts. Alternatively, perform the movement while travelling around in a circle, or while travelling anywhere in the hall or field.

Exercise 6.9	Travelling side squats (pulse-raising)

Purpose

This exercise primarily assists with raising the pulse and warming the muscles. If a reasonably wide stride is taken on the squat movement there may be some effective mobilisation benefits for the hips. In addition, the bending and straightening action of the knees will provide some benefit for this area. If the arms are used, there may be mobilisation benefits for the shoulder and elbow joints.

If performed with a deeper bend and greater travel, this exercise can be used in the main workout as a low impact exercise to improve cardiovascular fitness.

Starting position and instructions

- Start with the feet hip-width apart
- Commence by stepping one leg to the side and squatting the legs apart
- Repeat this action for the desired number of repetitions in a particular direction
- Reverse the movement and travel in the opposite direction
- If working in a circle, it can be performed while facing into the centre of the circle or with the back to the centre of the circle.

Coaching points

- Squat the legs progressively to a larger range of motion, but only through a range that feels comfortable and achievable
- Keep the hips facing forwards and avoid hollowing of the lower back by tightening the abdominal muscles
- Avoid locking the knees as the leg straightens
- Keep the back straight and the chest lifted

- Ensure the knees move in line with toes
- Take care not to squat too deeply –maintain a 90-degree angle at the knees.

Progressions/Adaptations

- Start with a static squat and progress to one small squat in each direction (right/left)
- Initially take smaller strides and progressively increase stride length to increase the range of motion
- Start more slowly and move at a progressively quicker pace
- Perform more repetitions in one direction to increase travel and raise the intensity
- Add movement of the arms, e.g. biceps curls, triceps extensions, chest press/shoulder press, to add variety and increase motor skills.

| Exercise 6.10 | Easy walk or box step (pulse-raising) |

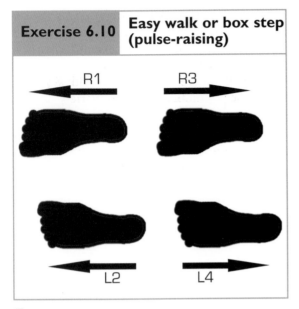

Purpose

This exercise primarily assists with raising the pulse and warming the muscles. If it is performed with a greater intensity (bending deeper) or with impact (jumping back instead of stepping back), it can effectively be used to improve cardiovascular fitness. It is also useful when introducing the circuit. It can be performed by participants while the teacher demonstrates a step-up movement.

Starting position and instructions

- Start with the feet hip-width apart
- Step forwards and take the weight onto the right leg
- Step the left leg forwards and level with the right leg
- Step the right leg backwards and take the weight onto the right leg
- Step the left leg back to the start position. At this point one can either tap the floor with the left foot and step forwards, repeating the sequence with a left leg lead (alternating box

step); or place the weight onto the left leg and step forwards, repeating the sequence on the right leg for the desired number of repetitions before changing legs.

Coaching points

- Take a large but comfortable step forwards with the legs
- Keep the hips facing forwards and avoid hollowing of the lower back by tightening the abdominal muscles
- Keep the knee joints unlocked and do not allow the knees to roll inwards
- Keep the chest lifted and body upright
- If impact is added, make sure the heels go down to cushion the movement.

Progressions/Adaptations

- Start with a smaller step and progressively increase step stride
- Move at a progressively faster tempo
- Bend deeper to add intensity
- Perform more repetitions with the same leg, leading to increased muscular endurance.

Add impact for cardiovascular training by either stepping forwards and jumping back instead of stepping; or jumping forwards instead of stepping and stepping only on the backward phase of the movement.

Exercise 6.11	Walking (pulse-raising)

Purpose

This exercise primarily assists with raising the pulse and warming the muscles. If it is performed with a greater intensity (larger strides to travel further) or with impact (skipping or jogging instead of walking) it can effectively be used to improve cardiovascular fitness.

Starting position and instructions

• Stand with the feet hip-width apart
• Walk forwards for the desired number of counts and then change direction or walk backwards for the desired number of counts.

Coaching points

• Take a large but comfortable step forwards with the leg
• Use heel–toe action when walking forwards
• Keep the hips facing forwards and avoid hollowing of the lower back by tightening the abdominal muscles
• Keep the knee joints unlocked and do not allow the knees to roll inwards.
• Keep the chest lifted and body upright
• If impact is added, make sure the heels go down to cushion the movement.

Progressions/Adaptations

• Start with a smaller step and progressively increase step stride
• Move at a progressively faster tempo
• Perform more repetitions in the same direction to assist those with limited motor skills
• Add impact for cardiovascular training by jogging forwards

• Travel the movement in different directions for variation. For example, forwards and backwards, around in a circle, or just free walking anywhere in the room
• Use with different arm lines or with shoulder and spine mobility to add variety to the warm-up
• Walk with the body low (Groucho Marx) for a few repetitions and/or raising the body up on the toes for a few repetitions.

PRE- AND POST-WORKOUT STRETCHING AND FLEXIBILITY EXERCISES

7

Points to consider when designing the stretching and flexibility part

- These stretches can be used for preparatory and post-workout maintenance stretching. However, it is important to consider the environmental temperature and possible interruptions to class flow if using floor-based stretches in the warm-up. It is essential that the benefits of the warm-up are not lost
- Specific stretches for the upper body can be performed in a seated or kneeling position as well as the standing position illustrated
- Developmental stretches are best performed in a more supportive position offering comfort and stability. Floor-based stretches are often more appropriate.

Exercise 7.1	Back of thigh stretch

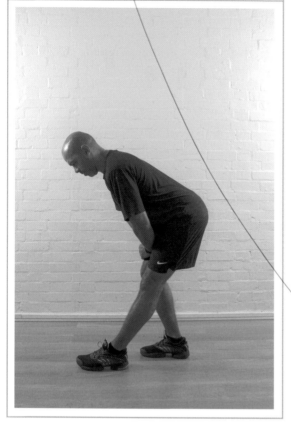

Purpose

This exercise lengthens and stretches the hamstring muscles at the back of the thighs, and also the buttock muscles (gluteals).

Starting position and instructions

- Stand with feet hip-width apart
- Step forwards with one leg, a shoulder-width stride
- Bend the knee of the back leg and place the hands at the top of the thigh of the bent knee
- Bend forwards from the hips and slide the hands down the thigh of the bent knee until

a mild tension is felt at the back of the thigh of the straight leg.

Coaching points

- Keep the weight-bearing knee joint slightly bent and ensure the knee joint does not roll inwards
- Only bend forwards to a point where a mild tension is felt at the back of the thigh
- Keep the knee of the straight leg fully extended, but not locked out
- Keep the hips square and pull the abdominals in to avoid hollowing the lower back
- Keep the spine long and the chest lifted
- Lift the buttocks higher and push them backwards to increase the stretch at the back of the thigh.

Progressions/Adaptations

- Start with a smaller range of motion by bending forwards only slightly
- Progress to lifting the buttocks higher and extending the straight leg
- Take a larger step forwards to increase the range of motion.

Exercise 7.2	Front of thigh stretch

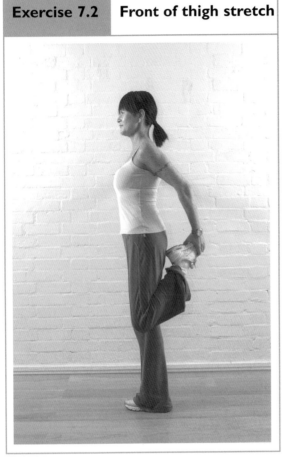

Purpose

This exercise lengthens and stretches the quadriceps muscles at the front of the thigh. If the hips are tilted forwards, it will also stretch the hip flexor muscles (iliopsoas).

Starting position and instructions

- Balance on one leg
- Raise the heel of the opposite leg towards the buttock cheek
- Use the hand to hold the leg and achieve a fuller range of motion – hold still.

Coaching points

- Keep the supporting knee joint unlocked
- Only lift the leg to a point where a mild tension is felt at the front of the thigh, do not overflex (bend) the knee
- Keep the hips facing forwards and avoid hollowing of the lower back by keeping the abdominal muscles pulled in tight
- Lift the heel towards the centre of the buttock cheeks – avoid taking the heel to the outside of the buttocks as this may stress the ligaments on the inside of the knee
- Tilt the hips slightly forwards
- Keep both knees in line with each other.

Progressions/Adaptations

- Start with a smaller range of motion by lifting the leg less high. A towel around the ankle can be used to hold the ankle if desired
- Keep the knee of the stretching leg slightly in front of the other knee to decrease the stretch
- Take the knee of the stretching leg slightly back, so that it is positioned to the side of, but slightly behind, the other knee to increase the stretch
- Progressively lift the heel closer towards the buttocks to achieve a greater range of motion
- Tilt the hips forwards to increase the stretch slightly
- Hold on to a wall or partner to assist balance
- Bend and straighten the knee of the supporting leg while performing the stretch to add variety and improve motor skills.

Exercise 7.3	Calf stretch

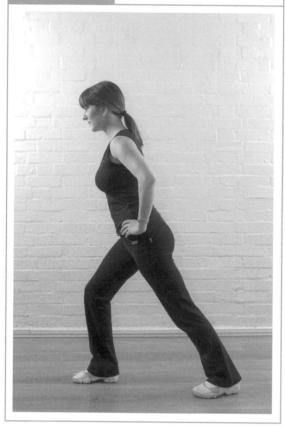

Coaching points

- Keep the front knee bent but do not let the knee roll inwards
- Keep the heel of the back foot facing forwards
- Keep the hips facing forwards and avoid hollowing of the lower back by tucking the buttock muscles under
- Keep a straight line through the body from the heel of the back foot through to the head. Take care not to bend forwards at the hip
- Keep the chest lifted and the abdominals pulled in.

Progressions/Adaptations

- For a smaller range of motion, only step the leg a short distance backwards
- Hold a wall or a partner to assist balance
- Combine with upper body stretches for variety, if motor skills allow
- Lean into a wall or partner while performing the stretch to increase the range of motion. Ensure correct alignment is maintained.

Purpose

This exercise lengthens and stretches the gastrocnemius and soleus muscles at the back of the lower leg.

Starting position and instructions

- Start with the feet hip-width apart
- Step the right leg backwards, as far as possible but keeping the heel of the back foot on the floor. Keep the left (front) knee bent.

Exercise 7.4	Inner thigh stretch

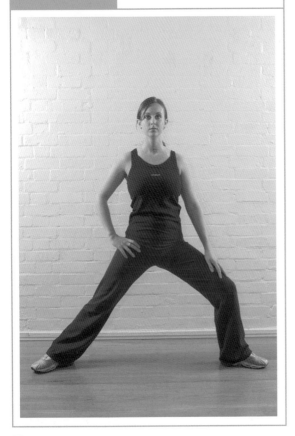

Purpose

This exercise lengthens and stretches the adductor muscles at the inside of the thigh.

Starting position and instructions

- Stand with the legs shoulder-width-and-a-half apart
- Bend the right knee, taking the body weight towards the right
- Keep the left knee straight but not locked
- Repeat on the other side to stretch the left adductor.

Coaching points

- Keep the knee joint of the weight-bearing leg unlocked, and the knee in line with toes over the ankle
- Step the legs further apart to increase the stretch of the inner thigh and groin
- Keep the hips facing forwards and avoid hollowing of the lower back by tucking the buttock muscles under
- Position the foot of the stretching leg in a comfortable position, ideally keeping the knees in line with the toes.

Progressions/Adaptations

- Start with a smaller range of motion, with the legs only a short distance apart
- Progress by stepping the legs wider apart, but only to a point where correct alignment of the knees can be maintained
- Tilt the pelvis sideways towards the weight-bearing knee to increase the stretch slightly
- Hold on to a wall to assist balance
- For those with greater motor skills, combine with upper body stretches to add variety
- Stretch both legs together by squatting with the knees turned out, using the arms to press the knees out to the side.

Exercise 7.5	Side stretch

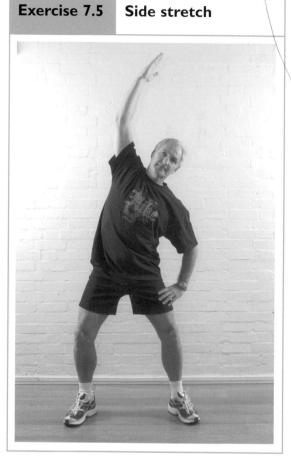

NB: this can be performed in a seated position and as a post-workout stretch.

Purpose

This exercise lengthens and stretches the muscles at the sides of the trunk and the back, the obliques and latissimus dorsi.

Starting position and instructions

- Stand with the feet shoulder-width-and-a-half apart, with the knees unlocked
- Place the right hand on the left hip to support the body weight
- Lift the left arm up and bend over slightly to the right side.

Coaching points

- Keep the knee joint of both legs slightly bent
- Emphasise lifting the body upwards rather than leaning too far over to the side
- Stretch only to a point where a mild tension is felt at the side of the trunk
- Keep the hips facing forwards and avoid hollowing of the lower back by tucking the buttock muscles under
- Keep the body weight equally placed between the two legs; avoid pushing the hip out to the side
- When bending to the side, move the body in a straight line and do not lean forwards or backwards
- Lift the ribcage upwards and create a gap between the pelvis and the ribs before bending to the side.

Progressions/Adaptations

- Start by only reaching the arm up and not bending over to the side. Alternatively, keep both hands on the hips and bend over to the side. This will decrease the stretch slightly and will take out any muscular work of the shoulder required to hold the arm up.
- Stretch the arm higher and bend over further to achieve a greater range of motion. Ensure the correct alignment of the spine is maintained.

NB: it is not advisable to perform this stretch with both arms out to the side. Firstly, this places a lot of unnecessary weight on the spine. Secondly, the muscles may not be able to relax and therefore may not stretch effectively.

| Exercise 7.6 | **Back of the upper arm stretch** |

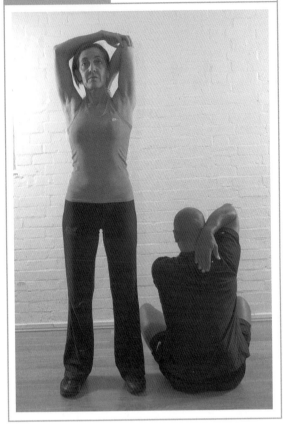

Note: this can be performed in a seated position and as a post-workout stretch. It can also be performed while bending the knees or walking around the room to maintain pulse-raising, if motor skills allow.

Purpose

This exercise lengthens and stretches the triceps muscles at the back of the upper arm.

Starting position and instructions

- Stand with the feet hip-width apart
- Place one hand in the centre of the back and

use the other arm to ease the arm further back – hold still.

Coaching points

- Keep the knee joint of both legs slightly bent.
- Keep the hips facing forwards and avoid hollowing of the lower back by tucking the buttock muscles under and pulling the abdominals in
- Stretch only to a point where a mild tension is felt at the back of the upper arm.

Progressions/Adaptations

- For people with less flexibility, start with the hand on the shoulder and use the opposite hand to raise the arm up slightly and through a smaller range of motion
- Progress by easing the arm further back and downwards into the position.
- Progress further by taking the other arm behind the back into a half-nelson position and attempting to reach the fingers of the stretching arm. This will stretch the deltoid muscles at the front of the shoulder
- Perform with a lower body stretch of the calves or adductors for variety, if motor skills allow.

Exercise 7.7	Chest stretch

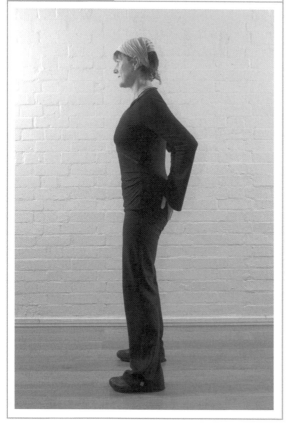

NB: this can be performed in a seated position and used for the post-workout stretch. It can also be performed while bending the knees or walking around the room to maintain pulse-raising, if motor skills allow.

Purpose

This exercise lengthens and stretches the muscles of the chest (pectorals).

Starting position and instructions

- Stand with the feet hip-width apart
- Take the hands backwards until a mild tension is felt at the front of the chest

- The hands can be placed on the buttocks or clasped together behind the back, whatever is most comfortable.

Coaching points

- Keep the knees unlocked
- Keep the elbows slightly bent
- Squeeze the shoulder blades together and lift the chest to increase the stretch
- Keep the hips facing forwards and avoid hollowing of the lower back by tucking the buttock muscles under and tightening the abdominal muscles.

Progressions/Adaptations

- Start with a smaller range of motion
- Move the arms progressively through a greater range of motion by linking the fingers and lifting the arms up slightly
- Taking the arms further back, allowing the hands to touch the buttocks and squeezing the shoulder blades together will also increase the stretch for the pectorals
- Perform with a lower body stretch of the calves or adductors to add variety, if motor skills allow.

| Exercise 7.8 | Middle back stretch | Exercise 7.9 | Side of trunk stretch |

Exercise 7.8 Middle back stretch

NB: this can be performed in a seated position for use in the post-workout stretch while bending the knees or walking around the room to maintain pulse-raising, if motor skills allow.

Purpose

This exercise stretches the muscles in the middle of the back, the trapezius.

Starting position and instructions

- Stand with feet shoulder-width-and-a-half apart
- Take both arms forwards, just below shoulder height, and link the fingers
- Round the shoulders slightly to feel a mild tension in the middle of the upper back.

Coaching points

- Keep knees unlocked and elbows slightly bent
- Keep the hips facing forwards and avoid hollowing of the lower back by tucking the buttock muscles under and tightening the abdominal muscles
- Round the shoulders slightly but without leaning forwards at the hip.

Progressions/Adaptations

- Start with a smaller range of motion, not rounding the shoulders so far
- Move the arms progressively through a greater range of motion by rounding the shoulders further
- Wrapping the arms around the body with the hands touching the back (hug yourself) will increase the stretch for the trapezius
- Perform with a lower body stretch of the calves or adductors to add variety, if motor skills allow.

Exercise 7.9 Side of trunk stretch

NB: this can be performed in a seated position and used for the post-workout stretch.

Purpose

This exercise lengthens and stretches the muscles at the sides of the trunk and the back, the obliques and latissimus dorsi.

Starting position and instructions

- Stand with the feet one-and-a-half times shoulder-width apart, with the knees unlocked
- Raise both arms above the head and interlink the fingers
- Keeping the shoulders relaxed and down, extend and lengthen the body upwards.

Coaching points

- Keep the knee joint of both legs slightly bent
- Emphasise lifting the body upwards
- Stretch only to a point where a mild tension is felt at the side of the trunk
- Keep the hips facing forwards and avoid hollowing of the lower back by keeping the abdominals pulled in tight
- Keep the shoulders relaxed
- Keep the body weight equally placed between the two legs.

Progressions/Adaptations

- For participants with lower motor skills, this exercise can be performed standing still
- Start by only reaching the arm up and not bending over to the side. Alternatively keep both hands on the hips and bend over to the side. This will decrease the stretch slightly and will take out any muscular work of the shoulder required to hold the arm up.

Exercise 7.10	Back of thigh stretch (lying)

Purpose

This exercise lengthens and stretches the hamstring muscles at the back of the thigh, and also the buttock muscles (gluteals).

Starting position and instructions

- Lie on the back with the knees bent and the feet firmly on the floor
- Raise one leg towards the chest and hold at the back of the thigh or calf, wherever is most comfortable
- Use the hand to support the leg and achieve a fuller range of motion; hold still
- To develop, allow the tension to ease and then use the hands to guide the leg into a larger range of motion.

Coaching points

- Keep the lower back on the floor
- Only lift the leg to a point where a mild tension is felt at the back of the thigh
- Aim to extend the knee fully on the stretching leg
- Keep the head and shoulders supported on the floor
- Keep the knee joint of the other leg bent.

Progressions/Adaptations

- Start with a smaller range of motion by lifting the leg less high, if necessary using a towel around the leg to hold it
- Keep the knee slightly bent if fully extending the knee is uncomfortable
- Progress to extending the knee straight and easing the leg closer to the chest.

| Exercise 7.11 | **Front of thigh stretch** |

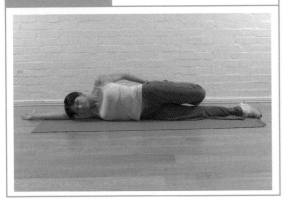

NB: this can be performed lying on one side or lying face down.

Purpose

This exercise lengthens and stretches the quadriceps muscles at the front of the thigh. If the hips are tilted forwards, it will also stretch the hip flexor muscles, the iliopsoas.

Starting position and instructions

- Lie either on the tummy or on one side
- Raise the heel of the one leg towards the centre of the buttock cheek
- Use the hand to hold the leg and achieve a fuller range of motion; hold still
- To develop, when the tension eases take the knee further back and press the hips forwards.

Coaching points

- Only lift the leg to a point where a mild tension is felt at the front of the thigh; do not overflex (bend) the knee
- Keep the back straight and abdominal muscles pulled in
- Keep the hips facing forwards and avoid hollowing of the lower back
- Lift the heel towards the centre of the buttock cheeks; avoid taking the heel to the outside of the buttocks, as this may stress the ligaments on the inside of the knee
- Tilt the hips slightly forwards
- Aim to keep both knees in line with each other.

Progressions/Adaptations

- It may be easier for less flexible participants to lie on their side. This allows the knee to be positioned slightly in front of the body and the range of motion to be smaller
- A towel can be used to hold the ankle and decrease the range of motion
- Lift the heel progressively closer towards the buttocks to achieve a greater range of motion
- Tilt the hips forwards to increase the stretch slightly
- Take the knee of the stretching leg slightly back, so that it is positioned to the side but slightly behind the other knee to increase the stretch.

Exercise 7.12	Calf stretch – seated

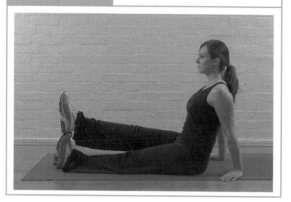

Purpose

This exercise lengthens and stretches the gastrocnemius and soleus muscles at the back of the lower leg.

Starting position and instructions

- Sit up straight with the legs in front of the body. If it is more comfortable to lean slightly backwards, the arms should be placed on the floor behind the body to support the body weight
- Place the heel of one foot over the toe of the other foot and use the top leg to ease the toes towards the body, stretching the calf muscle.

Coaching points

- Keep the knee joint of both legs unlocked
- Only move to a point where a mild tension is felt in the calf
- Keep the hips facing forwards and avoid hollowing of the lower back by pulling the abdominal muscles in tight
- Keep the shoulders relaxed and down.

Progressions/Adaptations

- Move through a smaller range of motion by only easing the foot a short distance towards the body
- Ease the toes closer to achieve a greater range of motion
- Use the hands to reach forwards and ease the foot towards the body

NB: this will only be achieved by participants who have flexible hamstrings.

- As a variation, lie down on the back to perform the same stretch. Keep the legs on the floor, not in the air.

| Exercise 7.13 | **Inner thigh stretch** |

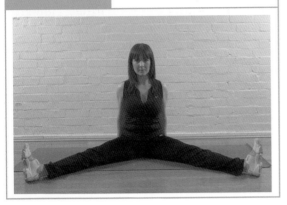

Purpose

This exercise lengthens and stretches the adductor muscles in the inner thighs.

Starting position and instructions

- Sit on the floor with either the soles of the feet together, or with the legs straddled out wide
- The hands can be placed on the floor behind the back to help maintain an upright position of the spine
- Flexible participants who are able to keep their spine upright can keep the hands in front of the body and on the floor.

Coaching points

- Keep the back straight and the chest lifted
- Visualise the vertebrae as bricks and the vertebrae discs as marshmallows to maintain an upright spine
- Aim to feel a mild tension in the inner thighs and groin
- Keep the hips facing forwards and avoid hollowing of the lower back
- Breathe comfortably.

Progressions/Adaptations

- Start with a smaller range of motion in the straddle position by taking the legs out less far. Progress by taking the legs wider apart
- Start with a smaller range of motion in the soles of feet together position by keeping the feet further away from the body and easing the knees only a small distance towards the floor. Progress by bringing the feet closer to the body and easing the knees further down towards the floor
- Both positions can be performed lying on the back

NB: if lying on the back with the legs straddled and raised in the air, ensure that the legs stay in line over the belly button and support the weight of the legs by holding the outside of the knees with the hands. This will allow the muscles to relax more easily.

- Another lying alternative is to bring the knees towards the armpits with the soles of the feet together or slightly apart, holding the ankles to ease the legs in further.

Exercise 7.14	Back of thigh stretch – seated

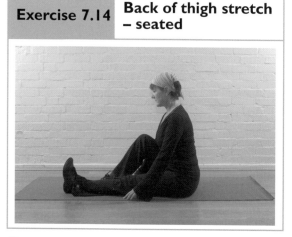

Purpose

This exercise lengthens and stretches the muscles at the back of the thigh (hamstrings).

Starting position and instructions

- Sit upright with one leg out straight in front of the body and the other leg out to the side
- Bend forwards from the hip to feel a stretch in the back of the thigh.

Coaching points

- For persons with less flexible hamstrings and who are less able to bend forwards from the hip, the hands can be behind the back to keep the spine supported
- Keep the knee of the stretching leg slightly bent
- Emphasise lifting the body upwards and stretch to a point where a mild tension is felt at the back of the thigh
- Keep the chest lifted and the abdominal muscles pulled in
- Ensure the other leg is in a comfortable position. Avoid the hurdle position as this may place stress on the ligaments at the inside of the knee joint.

Progressions/Adaptations

- Start by only bending a little way forwards
- Progress by bending over slightly further to achieve a greater range of motion
- Push the buttocks further backwards on the stretching leg to increase the stretch
- Both legs can be stretched at the same time if participants are sufficiently flexible. However, it should be noted that the range of motion will be limited to the range achievable by the less flexible muscle.

Exercise 7.15	Hip flexor stretch

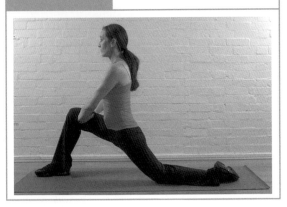

Purpose

This exercise lengthens and stretches the iliopsoas muscle which runs through to the front of the femur (thigh bone) from the pelvis and the lumbar spine.

Starting position and instructions

- Step one leg forwards into a lunge position with the foot flat on the floor
- Keep the other knee on the floor and press the hip forwards to feel a stretch through the hip
- The hands can be rested on the floor to assist balance; ideally keep the chest lifted.

Coaching points

- Keep the back straight
- Keep the hips facing forwards
- Stretch only to a point where a mild tension is felt
- Keep the knee of the front leg in line over the ankle
- Ensure the knee does not overshoot the toe.

Progressions/Adaptations

- Less flexible participants can perform this stretch standing up, with one leg back slightly and the hips tilted forwards. This can be progressed gradually by taking the leg further back and sinking the body weight down towards the floor
- This position can be progressed by initially taking the legs a smaller distance apart and gradually taking them to a further but comfortable distance apart.
- Tilt the pelvis forwards while performing the stretch to increase the range of motion slightly.

Exercise 7.16	**Outside of hip and thigh stretch**

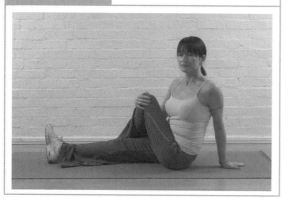

Purpose

This exercise lengthens and stretches the muscles at the sides of the hips and thighs, the abductors. It may also provide a stretch for the muscles at the sides of the back, and in the lower back (erector spinae).

Starting position and instructions

- Sit upright with both legs out in front of the body
- Bend the right knee and cross it over the left leg, placing the right foot on the floor by the side of the left knee
- Lift the chest up and twist the body towards the right, placing the left elbow against the right knee to ease the stretch further.

Coaching points

- Keep the spine upright
- Keep the hips facing forwards and avoid hollowing of the lower back
- Twist the body from the trunk, keeping the buttocks firmly placed on the floor
- Rotate around only as far as is comfortable.

Progressions/Adaptations

- Start with a smaller range of motion; do this by not twisting the body around so far. Move progressively to a greater range of motion by twisting further around and using the arm to ease the leg further away from the direction in which the body is turning.

Exercise 7.17	**Back stretch**

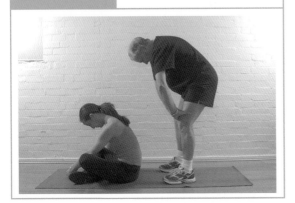

NB: this exercise can be performed in a standing position by leaning forwards, placing the hands on the knees and rounding the back and neck.

Purpose

This exercise lengthens and stretches the muscles of the back (erector spinae).

Starting position and instructions

- Sit upright with the legs crossed in front of the body
- Bend the body forwards and curl the spine over, lengthening the neck and the whole of the spine.

Coaching points

- Keep the spine curled over and relaxed
- Keep the buttock muscles firmly on the floor
- Keep the hands on the floor to support the weight of the body
- Only stretch to a point where a mild tension is felt.

Progressions/Adaptations

- Start with a smaller range of motion, by bending only a little way forwards
- Move progressively to a greater range of motion by bending further forwards. Participants who can bend forwards comfortably through a large range of motion can place their hands at the back of the head to increase the stretch in this area
- Have the legs crossed a further distance from the body if sitting cross-legged is not comfortable.

Stretching exercises using the step

Most upper body stretches can be performed in a seated position on the step. This can assist the performance of stretches in some individuals, by reducing the level of flexibility required in the hamstrings and erector spinae, which they would need to maintain an upright posture in a floor-seated position.

Exercise 7.18	**Chest (Pectorals)**

- In seated position, place hands at back end of the step and press chest forwards to stretch pectorals, keeping elbows unlocked
- Lying with back on the step, allow arms to drop to each side of the step.

Exercise 7.19	**Adductors: seated on step**

- Place soles of feet together
- Legs should be straddled
- Bend knees in a squat position and ease knees out using hands.

NB: sitting on the step will reduce the flexibility demanded from the hamstrings and erector spinae to maintain an upright position. The higher the step, the easier the stretch will be.

| Exercise 7.20 | **Adductors: seated on floor** |

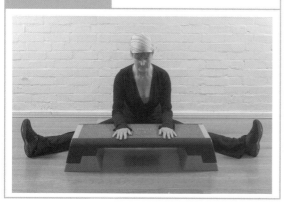

- Straddle legs with the ankles outside the step. Lean forwards towards the step and ease the body forwards to increase the stretch.

| Exercise 7.21 | **Hamstrings: seated on step** |

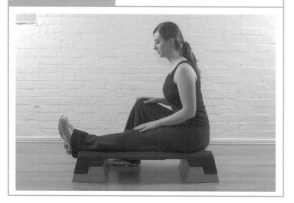

- With one leg resting across the length of the step, lean forwards into stretch
- Place bottom on the step with legs resting on the floor, one knee bent, and lean towards straight leg.

| Exercise 7.22 | **Hamstrings: seated on floor** |

- Place one foot on the step to increase the range of motion.

NB: sitting on the step will reduce the flexibility demanded from the hamstrings and erector spinae to maintain an upright position. The higher the step, the easier the stretch will be.

| Exercise 7.23 | **Hip flexor: kneeling on step** |

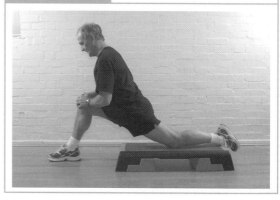

- One knee on the step, other leg lunges forwards on the floor. This position is more supportive, enhancing the stretch.

CIRCUIT TRAINING FOR CARDIOVASCULAR FITNESS

8

How should the complete session be structured?

Some circuit training programmes are designed primarily to improve cardiovascular fitness. This chapter discusses how to structure these sessions and how to monitor intensity. For a detailed outline of why cardiovascular training is important in general fitness, please refer to Chapter 1.

To specifically train to improve cardiovascular fitness, the session should comprise the components shown in Table 8.1.

Appropriate activities to re-warm the body and increase the intensity in preparation for cardiovascular training

The re-warmer component should commence with less intense versions of the activities to be performed in the main circuit. The intensity of each exercise will need to be progressively built up to the desired level. This can be achieved by starting with relatively small movements and gradually increasing the size of the movement. Progressively moving the centre of gravity in one or a combination of the following ways will

Table 8.1	The structure of a circuit to improve cardiovascular fitness
Warm-up	• mobility and pulse-raising activities • preparatory stretches
Main circuit: cardiovascular training (essential)	• re-warmer to raise the intensity (elevate heart rate into training zone – see pages 68–71) and introduce the exercises to be used in the circuit • maintenance of intensity (maintain heart rate within the recommended training zone). Providing intervals of higher-intensity exercises combined with lower-intensity exercises is ideal. • cool-down to lower intensity (lower the heart rate out of the training zone) and promote venous return.
Cool-down	• post-workout stretches (developmental and maintenance stretches) • relaxation activities (optional) • remobilise

increase intensity and build cardiovascular fitness:

- upwards (jumping)
- downwards (bending the knees)
- travelling direction (walking, running).

Other methods of building intensity include:

- increasing the speed of the movement
- using additional muscle groups (combining arm movements with leg work)
- lengthening levers (straight leg kicks instead of knee raises).

What activities are appropriate to train cardiovascular fitness in the main circuit?

Ultimately, a balanced combination of travelling movements, higher impact movements and lower impact stepping and bending movements are effective. This will bring about the desired training effect and maintain the safety of the workout by avoiding over-repetition of specific exercises.

A whole range of exercises appropriate to improve this component of fitness are listed at the end of this chapter.

What type of activities are appropriate to cool down and lower the intensity?

Exercises which progressively reduce the heart rate and breathing rate are safe and effective. Commencing with the larger activities used to maintain the intensity and gradually making the movements less intense will achieve the desired effect. This can be done by reducing

the number of jumping, travelling and deep bending movements, moving at a progressively slower pace, exerting less energy and utilising shorter levers (smaller kicks and arm movements).

How can I measure exercise intensity?

There are various ways of monitoring the intensity of an activity. Heart rate monitoring is one method. Maintaining the heart or pulse rate somewhere between 55 and 90 per cent of its maximum heart rate is suggested as an appropriate training range. An individual's maximum heart rate can be estimated by subtracting their age from 220. For example, a 30-year-old's maximal heart rate would be 190 beats per minute. The method used for calculating percentage of maximum heart rate is outlined in Table 8.2.

However, accurate heart rate monitoring is not easy. Lots of practice is needed to obtain a reasonably accurate reading. Frequently, the heart rate is miscalculated by missing counts at the start and finish of the count, hearing and counting echo beats within the count and/or counting the movements of the legs instead of the heart rate. NB: it is essential to keep the legs moving to avoid blood pooling.

It may therefore be appropriate to use an alternative method of monitoring intensity. Two alternative methods are the Talk Test and Rate of Perceived Exertion.

Talk test

Working to a level where one can breathe comfortably, rhythmically and hold a conversation while exercising is suggested to indicate an appropriate intensity. A guideline for using the Talk Test is provided in Table 8.3.

Table 8.2	Maximum heart rate and training zone for a 30-year-old

220 – 30 (age) = 190 beats per minute (maximum heart rate – MHR) 10 per cent of this maximum = 19 bpm
To calculate the training zone, multiply 19 (10 per cent of the MHR) by 5.5 (55 per cent) and 9.0 (90 per cent)

55 per cent of this maximum = 104 bpm (approx.)
(calculation: 10 per cent of maximal heart rate × 5.5)
90 per cent of this maximum = 171 bpm (approx.)
(calculation: 10 per cent of maximal heart rate × 9.0)

Therefore, the training zone for a 30-year-old would be between 104 and 171 bpm. They should work between this range in the main workout to improve their cardiovascular fitness.

Rate of Perceived Exertion (RPE)

Alternatively, Borg (1982) researched and developed the ratio RPE and CR10 category scales (6–20 and 0–10). An adaptation of the CR10 is outlined in Table 8.4. The scale provides a range of intensity levels from 0–10. An easy-to-remember verbal expression is used to suggest how the intensity of an activity is perceived by the performer. When the activity is perceived to be 'strong' (a rating between 4–7 on the scale), Borg suggests it should correspond to an appropriate intensity for improving cardiovascular fitness.

How accurate are these methods?

The accuracy of any of the aforementioned approaches is questionable. They should therefore only be used to provide a guideline as to how hard a person is working. It is perhaps advisable to use a combination of the methods and be constantly vigilant for signs of overexertion such as heavy breathing and excessive pallor or flushing of the skin.

Table 8.3	Using the Talk Test to monitor intensity	
Intensity level	**Talk Test response while performing an exercise**	**Action**
Too high	If one or only a few words can be spoken	Lower the intensity immediately
Too low	If a number of sentences can be spoken too comfortably	Increase the intensity
Appropriate	If a mild breathlessness is apparent at the end of speaking a couple of sentences	Maintain level of intensity

Table 8.4	Using Rate of Perceived Exertion to monitor intensity	
Scale	**Intensity**	**Verbal expression to describe the perceived intensity of activity**
0	Nothing at all	
0.5	Extremely light	Just noticeable
1	Very light	
2	Light	Weak
3	Moderate	
4	Somewhat heavy	
5	Heavy	Strong
6		
7	Very heavy	
8		
9		
10	Extremely heavy Maximal	Almost maximal Maximal

When might it be necessary to stop exercising?

Exercise should be stopped, and it is advisable to consult a doctor, if:

- normal co-ordination is lost while exercising
- dizziness occurs during exercise
- breathing difficulties are experienced
- tightness in the chest is experienced
- any other pain is experienced.

Summary of the guidelines for structuring the cardiovascular circuit

Re-warmer:
- Start at a lower intensity and progressively build to a higher intensity by bending deeper, jumping, and travelling further and more frequently
- Spend longer on this component with less fit groups to allow for a more progressive increase of heart rate
- Spend less time on this component with fitter participants who are able to build up to working at a higher intensity more rapidly.

Main circuit:
- Use exercises which utilise the large muscle groups to demand greater volumes of oxygen and create the desired effect
- Alter the stress on the joints by varying circuit stations. Alternate jumping exercise stations with stations that involve knee-bending and/or travelling and/or muscular strength and endurance exercises
- Utilise less frequent and shorter bursts of higher-intensity activities for less fit participants to enable them to work out safely and effectively

- Utilise frequent and longer bursts of more intense activities for fitter participants to make their heart work harder and challenge their cardiovascular system
- Use jumping movements sparingly with less fit persons who have a heavier body weight
- Spend longer on the whole circuit, possibly performing the circuit two to three times through, with fitter participants. This is dependent on the number of circuit stations used
- Spend comparatively less time on the circuit and at each individual circuit station for less fit participants.

Pulse-lowering:
- Start at a high intensity and progressively decrease the amount of jumping, travelling and depth of bending movements
- Spend longer on this component with less fit participants, allowing them a longer time to recover
- Spend less time on this component with fitter participants, who are generally able to recover more quickly.

CARDIOVASCULAR FITNESS EXERCISES

NB: all cardiovascular exercises will provide muscular endurance training for the lower body.

Purpose

This is a high-impact exercise for cardiovascular fitness.

Starting position and instructions

- Stand with feet hip-width apart
- Bend the knees and push through the thigh muscles to jump the legs to a wider, straddled position
- Raise the arms outwards to the sides of the body, in line with the shoulders, as the legs jump outwards
- Develop a rhythmic action.

Exercise 9.1	Jumping jacks

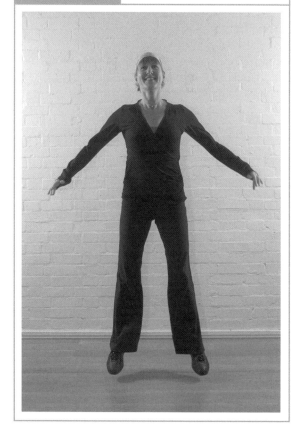

Coaching points

- Keep the knee joints unlocked
- Ensure the heels go down when landing
- Ensure the knees travel in line with the toes and over the ankles. Take care not to let the knees roll inwards
- Keep the elbows slightly bent throughout the movement
- Keep the abdominal muscles pulled in to avoid hollowing of the lower back
- Keep the hips facing forwards, the abdominals tight and the back straight.

Progressions/Adaptations

- To lower the impact, step the legs alternately out to the side without jumping. The

supporting knee must remain slightly bent and in line with the ankle. This exercise can be progressed by adding a jump in-between each alternate leg lunge (becomes high-impact when jumps added). Progressing to a higher jump and quicker movement will increase the intensity considerably
- Perform the jumping jacks at a slightly slower pace initially to lower intensity Increase the intensity by travelling the exercise forwards and backwards to move the resistance of the body across the force of gravity
- Increase the intensity further by progressing to a power jack. Achieve this by slowing down the jumping out movement and bending deeper, taking two counts, and performing two small jumps to draw the legs back together for two counts
- Add intensity by making the move explosive, leaping into the air, spreading arms and legs and landing in a tucked squat position ready to explode and jump upwards again.

Exercise 9.2	Jogging on the spot

Purpose

This is a high impact exercise for cardiovascular fitness.

Starting position and instructions

- Starting with the feet positioned slightly apart, commence jogging on the spot.

Coaching points

- Ensure the heels go down to the floor; this will maximise movement through the ankles and will prevent the calf muscles cramping (aim for a ball of the foot through to the heel landing)
- Land lightly
- Keep the knees unlocked and slightly soft throughout the movement
- Keep the hips facing forwards, the back straight and the abdominals pulled in
- If the arms are used, ensure they move in a controlled fashion and that the elbows remain unlocked
- If travelling the movement forwards, aim for a heel through to toe action of the foot to achieve a more natural running action.

Progressions/Adaptations

- To lower the impact, march or walk on the spot. (NB: it is essential that the feet land lightly to maintain marching as a low-impact exercise.)
- Start at a steadier pace and move through a smaller and lower range of motion where the feet lift only minimally from the floor
- Move at a progressively faster pace, and through a larger range of motion. Shifting the resistance of the body higher will increase the intensity of the movement
- Vary the speed of the movement. Try slow jogs where instead of moving to a single count, a half time count is used for each foot strike. Alternatively, speed the movement up to a sprint pace, or use a combination of slow and fast time, i.e. slow; slow; quick; quick; slow
- Travel the movement (shuttle runs or around the edge of the circuit). Shifting the body weight across the force of gravity in this way will increase the intensity of the movement.

Exercise 9.3	Spotty dogs

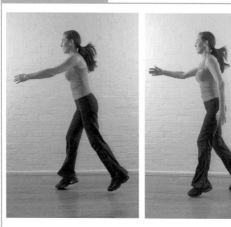

Purpose

This is a high-impact exercise for cardiovascular fitness.

Starting position and instructions

- Stand with the feet hip-width apart
- Bend the knees and push through the thighs to stride the legs alternately backwards and forwards
- Use the arms in opposition to the legs.

Coaching points

- Ensure the heels go down to the floor. Care should be taken not to force the heel of the back leg to the floor, unless it feels comfortable. This could potentially cause a ballistic stretch of the calf muscle, depending on the flexibility of the individual and the speed of the movement
- Stride the legs to a progressively larger range of motion, but only move through a range of motion that feels comfortable
- Keep the hips facing forwards and avoid hollowing of the lower back by tightening the abdominal muscles

- Keep both knees unlocked. This will avoid placing any stress on the cruciate ligaments, which help to stabilise the knee joints
- If the arms are used, ensure all movements are controlled and keep the elbows unlocked.

Progressions/Adaptations

- To lower the impact, step alternate legs backwards, keeping the weight-bearing knee slightly bent. Impact can be added and the intensity progressed in this variation by adding a jump as alternate legs lunge back. This will increase the intensity considerably
- Start with smaller strides and increase to a larger range of motion by increasing stride length
- Move at a progressively quicker pace
- Vary the speed of the movement. Moving more slowly and bending the knees deeper will vary the movement to a power lunge and will increase the intensity. Alternatively, combine some slow and some quicker-paced moves for power and speed, i.e. slow; slow; quick; quick; quick; quick.

Exercise 9.4	Leg kicks

Purpose

This is a high-impact cardiovascular exercise.

Starting position and instructions

- Stand with the feet hip-width apart.
- Hop on the right leg and at the same time kick the left leg forwards, to the side, or back
- Repeat this action, hopping on the left leg and kicking the right leg forwards, or to the side, or backwards.

Coaching points

- Keep the weight-bearing knee joint unlocked
- Take care not to lock the knee as the leg kicks forwards, sideways or backwards.
- Ensure the heel goes down as the foot lands. Soften the knee and take care not to let the knee roll inwards
- Keep the hips facing forwards and avoid hollowing of the lower back by keeping the abdominal muscles pulled in tight, the buttocks tucked under and the chest lifted.

Progressions/Adaptations

- For a low-impact exercise, leave out the hop (i.e. step and kick). Bend the knee of the weight-bearing leg to keep some intensity
- Start with a smaller hop and a lower kick
- Progress to a larger hop and a progressively higher kick of the leg
- Move forwards and/or backwards to shift the body weight across the force of gravity
- Vary the speed of the movement by performing some slower and quicker kicks
- Add variety by kicking the legs to the side of the body or behind the body
- Perform without a jump but lifting the legs higher to replicate a kick boxing movement. The body will need to lean slightly to compensate for the slightly higher movement of the legs. The abdominals must remain strong throughout
- Perform a variety of front, side and back kicks together as a kicking sequence, adding arm punches for further variety.

Exercise 9.5	Side shuffles/gallops

Purpose

This is a high-impact travelling exercise for cardiovascular fitness.

Starting position and instructions

- Stand with the feet hip-width apart
- Commence a sideways gallop to the right for the desired number of repetitions
- Return to the left with the same movement.

Coaching points

- Keep the knees slightly soft and unlocked.
- Ensure the heel goes down as the foot lands – take care not to just land on the ball of the foot
- Take care not to let the knees roll inwards
- Keep the hips facing forwards and avoid hollowing of the lower back
- Keep the abdominal muscles pulled in tight, the buttocks tucked under, the chest lifted and the shoulders back.

Progressions/Adaptations

- To lower the impact, walk to the side
- Start with less travel and progress by travelling further
- Start at a slower pace. Progress by galloping with more momentum and pace
- Stop before changing direction and returning the gallop to the start position
- Add variety by galloping in a circle (right leg leads) for the desired number of counts, pivot to face the back of the room and gallop in the same direction for further repetitions but with the left leg leading. Repeat
- Gallop from side to side mimicking a ball bouncing or high blocking action with the arm for sports such as basketball or netball.

Exercise 9.6	Tuck jumps

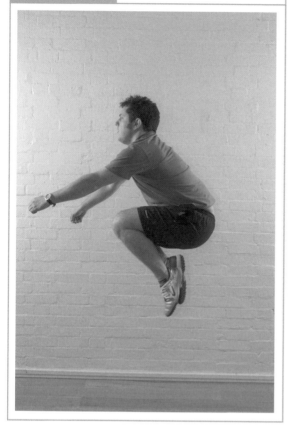

Purpose

This exercise will assist with the improvement of cardiovascular fitness. This movement is incredibly high-impact and explosive. It should only be used for fitter groups, and the repetitions limited to avoid strain.

Starting position and instructions

- Start with the feet hip-width apart
- Bend the knees and push through the thigh muscles to jump upwards
- The knees should move to the front of the chest
- Perform for the desired number of repetitions.

Coaching points

- Keep the knee joints unlocked
- Ensure the heels go down when landing
- Keep the elbows slightly bent throughout the movement
- Keep the hips facing forwards.

Progressions/Adaptations

- Start with a smaller tuck by pushing less forcefully through the thigh muscles
- Increase the height of the jump and the overall intensity of the movement
- Travel the movement
- Perform at a faster pace.

Exercise 9.7	Cossack squat kicks

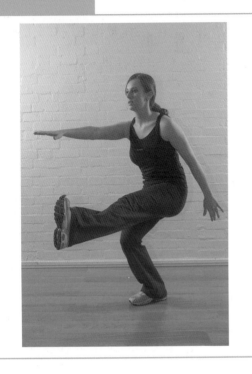

Purpose

This is a high-impact exercise for cardiovascular fitness.

Starting position and instructions

- Stand with the feet hip-width apart
- Squat down and kick the right leg out in front. Return from the squat bringing the leg in to the start position. Repeat with the left leg kicking
- Repeat this action, squatting and kicking alternate legs out.

Coaching points

- Keep the weight-bearing knee joint unlocked
- Take care not to lock the knees when returning from the squat or kicking
- Ensure the heel goes down as the foot lands. Soften the knee and take care not to let the knee roll inwards
- Keep the hips facing forwards and avoid hollowing of the lower back by keeping the abdominal muscles pulled in tight, the buttocks tucked under and the chest lifted.

Progressions/Adaptations

- To add impact, jump into squat position
- Start with a smaller hop and kick to a lower height
- Progress to a larger squat and a higher kick
- Travel the movement forwards and/or backwards
- Vary the speed of the movement by performing some slower kicks and some quick kicks.

Exercise 9.8	Leg side swings/ pendulums

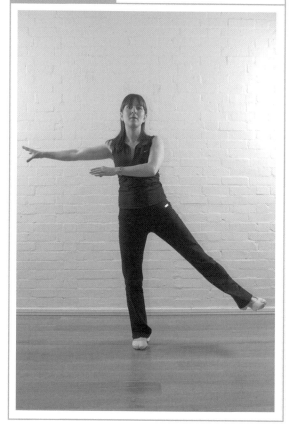

Purpose

This is a high-impact exercise for cardiovascular fitness. It can also be performed without impact (see photo).

Starting position and instructions

- Stand with the feet hip-width apart
- Hop on the right leg and at the same time kick the left leg out to the side, rocking and leaning the body towards the right
- Repeat this action, hopping on the left leg, kicking the right leg to the side and leaning the body towards the left
- Develop a rocking, swinging-type motion.

Coaching points

- Keep the weight-bearing knee joint unlocked
- Ensure the heel goes down as the foot lands. Soften the knee and take care not to let the knee roll inwards
- Keep the hips facing forwards and avoid hollowing of the lower back
- Keep the abdominal muscles pulled in tight, the buttocks tucked under, the chest lifted and the shoulders back.

Progressions/Adaptations

- To perform as a low-impact move, leave out the hop (i.e. the step and side kick). Bend the knee of the weight-bearing leg to maintain some intensity
- Start with a smaller hop and kick the legs sideways to a lower height
- Progressively increase to a larger hop, with more momentum and a higher kick to the side
- Travel the movement forwards and/or backwards to shift the body weight across the force of gravity
- Vary the speed of the movement by performing some slow and some quick movements, i.e. rock; rock hold right; rock; rock hold left.

| Exercise 9.9 | **Leg curls with bicep curls and hopscotch** |

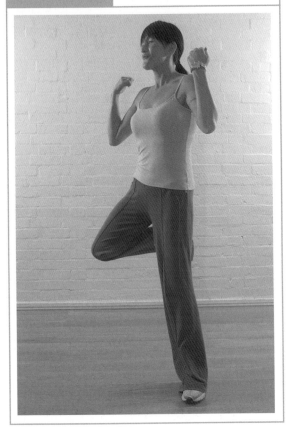

Purpose

This exercise will improve cardiovascular fitness if performed with a deep bend or a jump.

Starting position and instructions

- Start with the feet hip-width apart
- Step out to the right and transfer the weight over to the right, kicking the left heel towards the buttocks
- Step the left leg down and transfer the weight over to the left leg, kicking the right heel to the buttocks
- As the legs lift and lower, perform biceps

curling movements at the elbow or tap the heel behind the back
- Perform these alternating leg curls for the desired number of repetitions.

Coaching points

- Take large but comfortable strides
- Keep the hips facing forwards and avoid hollowing of the lower back by tightening the abdominal muscles
- Ensure the knee joint remains unlocked when landing
- Ensure the knees move in line with the toes and do not roll inwards
- Keep the back straight and the chest lifted
- Keep the movement controlled, smooth and not jerky
- If impact is added, make sure the heels go down to cushion the movement.

Progressions/Adaptations

- Start with a smaller stride and progressively increase stride length but ensure the distance is comfortable and correct alignment is maintained
- Move at a progressively quicker pace
- Bend deeper to promote greater pulse-raising
- Travel the movement forwards and backwards. This will add intensity because the body weight is being shifted across gravity. Progress further by travelling a greater distance in each direction
- Perform two or more leg curls to the same side. This requires slightly greater muscular endurance and will vary choreography.

Exercise 9.10	Knee lifts and arm pull-downs

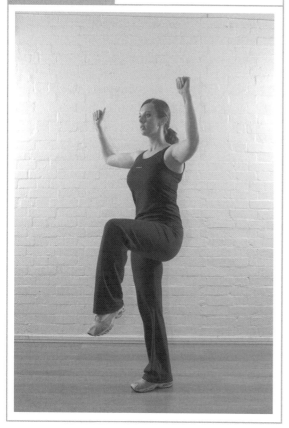

Purpose

This exercise will improve cardiovascular fitness. It can be performed with or without impact (jumping).

Starting position and instructions

- Start with the feet hip-width apart
- Step and shift the weight onto the right leg, lifting the left knee to hip height
- Step and shift the weight onto the left leg, lifting the right knee to hip height
- As the knee lifts, pull the arms down from above the head, raise the arms again until the other knee raises, then pull the arms down again
- Perform these alternating knee raises for the desired number of repetitions.

Coaching points

- Take comfortable strides
- Keep the hips facing forwards and avoid hollowing of the lower back by tightening the abdominal muscles
- Keep the knee joints unlocked and ensure the knees stay in line with the toes
- Lift the leg only to a height where an upright spine alignment can be maintained
- Keep the chest lifted and do not allow the body to bend forwards as the leg lifts
- If the exercise is used for cardiovascular training, and impact is added, make sure the heels go down to cushion the movement.

Progressions/Adaptations

- Start by lifting the leg only to a small height and progressively lift the leg higher
- Bend the weight-bearing leg a little deeper to add intensity
- Move at a slightly quicker pace
- Turn the movement in a circle (or as described for leg curls, see p. 65). This will add variety and challenge motor skills
- Perform two or more repetitions on the same side. This requires greater muscular endurance
- Travel the movement forwards and backwards to achieve a greater pulse-raising effect. Increase this further by performing a greater number of repetitions in one direction
- Increase intensity by adding impact to shift the resistance of the body upwards against gravity
- Perform four or more repetitions on each side and travel the movement in the direction that the knee is lifting.

Exercise 9.11	**Squats with arm circles (and squat jumps)**

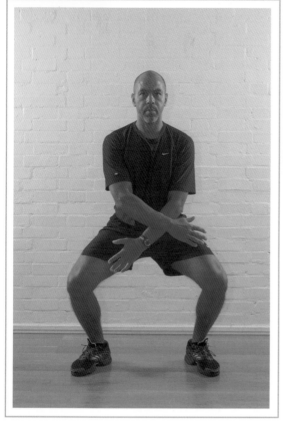

Purpose

This exercise will help to improve cardiovascular fitness.

Starting position and instructions

- Start with the feet hip-width-and-a-half apart.
- Bend and straighten the legs in a rhythmic fashion and circle the arms in front of the body at the same time.

Coaching points

- Squat the legs to a larger range of motion, but only move through a range of motion that feels comfortable and achievable
- Keep the hips facing forwards and avoid hollowing of the lower back by tightening the abdominal muscles
- Avoid locking the knees as the leg straightens
- Keep the back straight and the chest lifted
- Ensure the knees move in line with toes and over the ankles
- Take care not to squat too deeply – maintain a 90-degree angle at the knees.

Progressions/Adaptations

- Start with a static squat and leave out the arm movements
- Start slower and move at a progressively quicker pace
- Add impact by jumping in the air after every fourth bend
- Make the move plyometric (explosive) by jumping into the air after every squat
- Travel the movement to the side for the desired number of repetitions and then travel back.

Exercise 9.12	Shuttle walks, runs, sprints or hops

NB: all the movements can be performed statically at first and travel progressively. A skipping rope can be used if desired. Alternatively, a weighted sack can be dragged to make the exercises harder. Gymnastic crash mats can be used to run on; these will also add intensity to the movement and require greater power from the thigh muscles.

Purpose

This exercise assists with the improvement of cardiovascular fitness.

Starting position and instructions

- Stand with the feet hip-width apart
- Walk, jog, sprint or hop on one leg in a forward direction to a designated point
- Turn round and walk, jog or sprint back to the original point. If hopping, use the other leg
- A number of cones can be laid out and each one walked to and from in turn.

Coaching points

- Take a large but comfortable step forwards
- Heel–toe action when walking forwards
- Keep the hips facing forwards and avoid hollowing of the lower back by tightening the abdominal muscles
- Keep the knee joints unlocked and do not allow the knees to roll inwards (especially when hopping)
- Keep the chest lifted and the body upright
- Make sure the heels go down when jogging, hopping or skipping.

Progressions/Adaptations

- Move at a progressively quicker tempo
- Add impact by skipping, jogging or sprinting forwards
- Add impact and intensity by hopping the movement.

Exercise 9.13	Grapevine

Purpose

This exercise primarily assists with raising the pulse and warming the muscles. If it is performed with a greater intensity (bending deeper or travelling further) or with impact (hopping through the movement) it can effectively be used to improve cardiovascular fitness.

Starting position and instructions

* Stand with the feet hip-width apart
* Step the left foot out to the left side
* Cross-step the right leg behind the left leg and further towards the left direction, creating a small rotation of the body
* Step the left foot out to the left and place the foot or jump
* The movement can then either be repeated travelling to the left, or travelling back to the right leading with the right leg.

Coaching points

* Take a large but comfortable step to the side
* Keep the hips facing forwards and avoid hollowing of the lower back by tightening the abdominal muscles
* Keep the knee joints unlocked and do not allow the knees to roll inwards
* Keep the chest lifted and the body upright
* If impact is added for cardiovascular training, make sure the heels go down to cushion the movement.

Progressions/Adaptations

* Start with a smaller step and progressively increase step stride

* Move at a progressively quicker tempo
* Bend deeper to add intensity
* Perform more repetitions in the same direction to increase travel and shift the centre of gravity further
* Add impact for cardiovascular training by either hopping through the movement or jumping at the end
* Add a quarter-turn on the jump and repeat the sequence in a box shape
* Add a half-turn on the jump and perform the left-led grapevine facing the back wall. Repeat in order to return to face forwards.

Exercise 9.14	Squats, thrusts and burpees

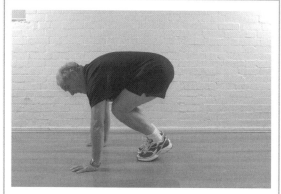

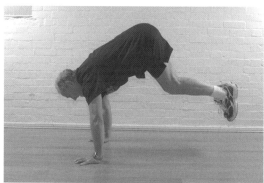

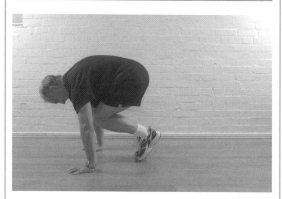

Purpose

These exercises will help to improve cardiovascular fitness. They are all very high-intensity and potentially controversial; they should therefore only be performed by fitter participants who can maintain accurate exercise technique.

Starting position and instructions

Squat thrust

- Start with the hands on the floor and the feet hip-width-and-a-half apart.
- Jump both legs back to an extended position (press-up position). Jump the legs back in again.

Alternate squat thrusts

Jump alternate legs back to lower the load (marginally) on the upper body.

Burpees

As for squat thrust, but on completion of a full squat thrust movement, jump into the air explosively. Repeat for desired number of repetitions.

Coaching points

- Keep the hips square and avoid hollowing of the lower back by tightening the abdominal muscles
- Avoid locking the knees as legs straighten
- Keep the back and the body straight
- Ensure the knees move in line with toes and over the ankles
- Take care not to squat too deeply – maintain a 90-degree angle at the knees
- Ensure the heels go down after the explosive

jumping phase of the burpee and soften the knees to absorb impact.

Progressions/Adaptations

- Start with back lunges, progress to double leg jumping forwards and backwards. Start slower and move at a progressively faster pace.
- Perform the movement with the hands on a bench or step initially, progressively lowering the movement to the floor.
- Progress steadily to burpees only when the other exercises can be executed safely.

Exercise 9.15	Continuous broad jumps and jumps forward and back

Purpose

These exercises will help to improve cardiovascular fitness. They are all very high-intensity and should therefore only be performed by fitter participants who can maintain accurate exercise technique.

Starting position and instructions

Broad jumps

- Start with the feet hip-width apart
- Jump forwards as far as you can, recover and jump forwards again.

Forwards and back jumps

- As above, but jump forwards a smaller distance and perform a recovery jump back to the start position.

Repeat either of the above exercises for the desired number of repetitions.

Coaching points

- Keep the hips square and avoid hollowing of the lower back by tightening the abdominal muscles
- Keep the back and the body straight
- Ensure the knees move in line with the toes and over the ankles
- Ensure the heels go down after each jump
- Soften the knees to absorb impact when landing
- Take care not to lock the knees.

Progressions/Adaptations

- Start with smaller jumps forwards and backwards
- Move at a progressively quicker pace and jump further
- Perform the exercises on a gymnastics mat to add intensity.

Exercise 9.16	Split jumps with and without arm punching

Purpose

This is a high-impact exercise for cardiovascular fitness.

Starting position and instructions

- Stand with the feet hip-width apart
- Bend the knees and push through the thigh muscles to jump the legs to a wider straddled position
- The arms raise outwards to the sides of the body, in line with the shoulders, as the legs jump outwards
- Jump the legs back in
- Then jump one leg forwards and one leg backwards ('spotty dog' action). The arms follow the same line of movement. Return to the start position
- Repeat above, performing one jump jack alternated with a spotty dog
- Develop a rhythmic action.

Coaching points

- Keep the knee joints unlocked
- Ensure the heels go down when landing
- Ensure the knees travel in line with the toes and over the ankles. Take care not to let the knees roll inwards
- Keep the elbows slightly bent throughout the movement
- Keep the abdominal muscles pulled in to avoid hollowing of the lower back
- Keep the hips facing forwards, the abdominals tight and the back straight.

Progressions/Adaptations

- To lower the impact, step the legs alternately out to the side and then backwards without jumping. The supporting knee must remain slightly bent and in line with the ankle. This exercise can be progressed by adding a jump in-between each alternate leg lunge (becomes high-impact when jumps added). Progressing to a higher jump and quicker movement will increase the intensity considerably
- Perform at a slower pace initially to lower intensity
- Leave out the arms to reduce complexity
- Add motor skills by punching the arms forwards instead of following the natural line of the movement
- Increase the intensity further by progressing to a power jack and/or power/explosive spotty dog movement. Achieve this by slowing down the jumping movements and bending deeper.

Exercise 9.17	Basic step/ V-step/Turn step

[a]

Left up 2   Right up 1

Left down 4 and tap to change lead leg   Start Right down 3

[b]

Left up 2   Right up 1

Left down 4 and tap to change lead leg   Start Right down 3

[c]

Left 2   Right 1

Left 5

Right 6

Right 3 Left 4 tap (turn to face right)   Left 7 Right 8 tap (turn to face left)

Purpose

These exercises can be used to improve cardiovascular fitness.

Starting position

- Stand with both feet hip-width apart.

Basic step (a)

- Step the right leg onto the step and bring the left leg up to meet it

- Step the right leg back down to the floor and bring the left leg back down to meet it
- Tap to change to a left leg lead when desired.

V-step (b)

- Step the feet out wide to each edge of the step, right foot to right edge and left foot to left edge
- Step the feet back down to the floor, hip-width apart (right foot then left foot)
- Tap to change to a left leg lead.

Turn step (c)

- As V-step, but turn the body in the direction of the movement.

Coaching points

- Keep the knee joints unlocked
- Keep the back straight and the abdominals pulled in
- Keep the hips facing forwards and fully extend the hip and knee
- Place the whole foot on the step and stay close to the step
- Keep the knees in line with the toes. Take care not to let the knees roll inwards
- Turn step only: turn the body prior to placing the foot on the step to avoid strain on the knee.

Progressions/Adaptations

- Start with slow time movement
- Progress by working to normal time
- Progress further by making each movement a run up onto the step
- Use different arm lines to add variety
- Jump and hold the legs in the V-step position (two counts) and step down to increase impact and intensity.

Exercise 9.18	Up & tap/Up & knee/ Up & curl/Up & raise side/Up & glute raise

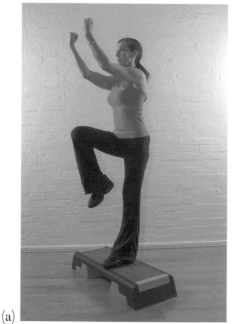

(a)

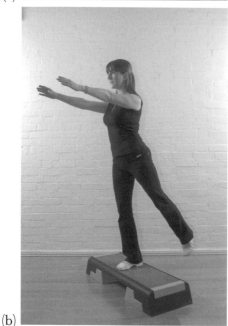

(b)

Purpose

These exercises can be used to train and improve cardiovascular fitness.

Starting position

• Stand with feet hip-width apart on the floor.

Up & tap

• Step the right foot onto the step and tap the step with the left leg, step down left, down right
• Repeat with the left leg leading.

Up & knee

• As above, but lift the knee to hip-height instead of tapping the step (see photo 9.18a).

Up & curl

• As above, but curl the heel towards the buttocks.

Up & raise side

• As above, but take the leg out towards the side.

Up & glute raise

• As above, but take the leg behind (see photo 9.18b).

Coaching points

• Keep the knee joints unlocked
• Keep the spine neutral and engage abdominals
• Keep the hips facing forwards and fully extend the hips and knees
• Place the whole foot on the step and stay close to the step

• Keep the knees in line with the toes. Take care not to let the knees roll inwards.

Progressions/Adaptations

• Start with slow time movement; progress by working to normal time
• Use different arm lines to add variety
• Perform a combination of the movements to challenge motor skills
• Travel the movement to the side of the step or bench
• Repeat the move for a specified number of counts each side to increase muscular endurance
• To add impact, jump up once the foot is placed on the step.

Exercise 9.19	Lunges (side and rear)

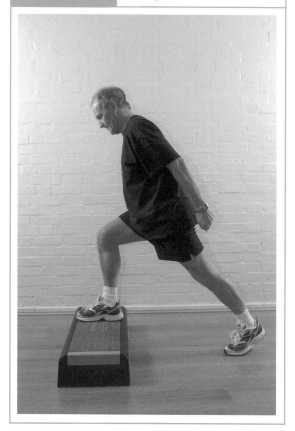

Purpose

This exercise can be used to train and improve cardiovascular fitness.

Starting position and instructions

- Stand on top of the step
- Lunge alternate legs off the step, right then left (either off the back or out to each side).

Coaching points

- Keep the knee joints unlocked and the whole foot on the step

- Keep the spine neutral and engage abdominals
- Keep knees in line with the toes and over the ankles, not letting the knees roll inwards
- Keep the hips facing forwards
- Tap the floor with the toe only. Do not transfer the weight of the body onto the lunging leg.

Progressions/Adaptations

- Start with a smaller lunge, just tapping the foot
- Progress by adding a rebound and jump between each lunge
- Move at a slightly quicker pace
- Perform a higher number of repetitions of lunges on the same leg to increase muscular endurance.

Exercise 9.20	Power squats

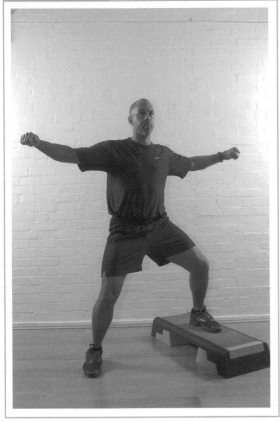

NB: this exercise can be performed on the floor without a step.

Purpose

This exercise will elevate and maintain the heart rate.

Starting position and instructions

- Stand on top of the step
- Step one leg out to the side in a squatting position. The other leg should stay in contact with the step

- Push through the thigh, and lift the body back onto the step and into the starting position
- Repeat, moving to the other side.

Coaching points

- Squat the legs to a comfortable range of motion
- Ensure the knees move in line with the toes and over the ankles
- Do not let the knees roll inwards
- Keep the hips facing forwards and avoid hollowing the lower back
- Avoid locking the knees as the leg straightens
- Keep the abdominals pulled in
- The whole foot should be on the step.

Progressions/Adaptations

- Start with a smaller and slower movement
- Move at a progressively quicker pace and make the movement larger
- Perform more repetitions on each side to increase muscular endurance
- Add a movement of the upper body (and weights, if fitness allows), i.e. a biceps curl or shoulder press
- Add a leg raise, leg curl or knee lift in-between each squat.

NB: these exercises can be used throughout the warm-up to introduce participants to movement patterns used in the main session, and to assist with mobility.

Exercise 9.21 (arm line) – Biceps curl

- Keeping the elbows pressed into the sides of the body, raise the forearm and curl the hands towards the shoulders in an arc-like motion. Return arms to sides without locking the elbows.

Exercise 9.22 (arm line) – Lateral raise

- Starting with the arms at the side of the body, raise the arms sideways until they are level with the shoulder
- Keep the elbows unlocked and the shoulders relaxed and down.

Exercise 9.23 (arm line) – Breaststroke

- Move the arms in a breaststroke swimming action either in front of the body or above the head
- Keep the shoulders relaxed and the elbows unlocked.

Exercise 9.24 (arm line) – Shoulder press

- Start with the arms bent and the hands level with the shoulders
- Extend the arms above the head and return to start position
- Keep the shoulders relaxed and the elbows unlocked.

Exercise 9.25 (arm line) – Front raise

- Start with the arms by the side of the body
- Raise the arms forwards in front of the body to shoulder height and lower again
- Keep the elbows slightly bent.

Exercise 9.26 (arm line) – Pec dec

- Start with the arms at shoulder height and the elbows bent, knuckles facing upwards
- Squeeze the arms together in front of the body and back to shoulder height
- Take care not to fling the arms too far back.

Exercise 9.27 (arm line) – Triceps kickback

- Start with the hands close to the armpits and the elbows pointing backwards
- Extend the lower arms out behind the back
- Do not lock the elbows
- Return the arms to a bent position
- Keep the arms back and only move the lower arm.

CIRCUIT TRAINING FOR MUSCULAR STRENGTH AND ENDURANCE

10

Some circuit training programmes are designed specifically to train only muscular strength and endurance. This chapter provides guidelines for structuring a muscular strength and endurance circuit. For a detailed outline of why muscular strength and endurance are important in general fitness please refer to Chapter 1.

What type of muscle work is most appropriate?

Activities that require the specific muscles and muscle groups to contract and work through a full range of motion, shortening and lengthening (isotonic movements) are most effective. Exercises that require the muscle to contract through a smaller range of motion or those which require the muscle to contract without the muscle lengthening and shortening (isometric contractions) are less effective. Some of the advantages and disadvantages of these two types of muscle work are outlined in Table 10.2.

Table 10.1	Session structure for a muscular strenth and endurance bias circuit
Warm-up	• mobility and pulse-raising activities • preparatory stretches • re-warm specific to the circuit to be performed. Allow time to introduce circuit exercises as necessary
Main circuit	• specific exercises targeting all major muscle groups to achieve a balanced whole body approach, with or without equipment (see Chapter 11 for example exercises)
Cool-down	• cooling down exercises. These exercises may actually need to re-warm the body prior to stretching • post-workout stretches (inclusion of developmental stretches will improve flexibility) • relaxation activities (optional) • remobilise

Table 10.2	Advantages and disadvantages of isotonic and isometric muscle work
Isotonic muscle work	**Isometric muscle work**
Strengthens the muscle through a full range of motion	Strengthens the muscle only in one position
Related to our daily activities	Most appropriate when moving the joint would cause injury (i.e. injury rehabilitation)
Requires the recruitment of a large proportion of muscle fibres and nerves	Requires the recruitment of only the specific muscle fibres to hold the position
	Can potentially elevate blood pressure
	Can cause participants to hold their breath

How should we train to improve muscular strength and endurance?

Training methods to improve muscular strength and endurance are discussed in greater detail in Chapter 11. A range of appropriate exercises to work the individual muscles are outlined in Table 10.3. Others exercises are detailed at the end of this chapter.`

Table 10.3	Joint actions in which the major muscle groups contract concentrically, and an example of exercises to work this muscle			
Muscle name	Anatomical position	Joints crossed	Prime action when contracting concentrically	Exercise
Gastrocnemius	Calf muscle	Knee and ankle	Plantarflexion – pointing the toe or rising onto the ball of the foot	Calf raise (11.24)
Soleus	Calf muscle	Ankle	As above – with knee bent	Calf raises (11.24) but with knee bent
Tibialis anterior	Front of shin bone	Ankle	Dorsiflexion of the ankle – lifting the toe up towards the knee with the heel on the floor	Toe tapping (11.21)
Hamstrings	Back of the thigh	Knee and hip	Flexion of the knee – lifting the heel towards the buttocks	Hamstring curls (11.16)
Quadriceps	Front of the thigh	Knee and hip	Extension of the knee – straightening the knee	Back squat (11.29) Dumbbell lunge (11.25) Dead-lift (11.22)
Gluteus maximus	Buttock	Hip	Extension of the hip – lifting the leg out straight behind the body	Rear leg raises Dead-lift (11.22) Dumbbell lunge (11.25)
Iliopsoas (hip flexor)	Front of hip	Hip	Flexion of the hip – lifting the knee to the chest	Knee lifts (6.6)
Abductors	Outside of hip and thigh	Hip	Abduction of the leg – taking the leg out to the side of the body	Side leg raises
Adductors	Inside thigh	Hip	Adduction of the hip – taking the leg across the front of the body	Side lying inner thigh raises Supine lying leg scissors

Table 10.3	Joint actions in which the major muscle groups contract concentrically, and an example of exercises to work this muscle cont.			
Rectus abdominis	Abdominals (front)	Spine	Flexion of the spine – bending the spine forwards	Sit-ups/curl-ups (11.1) Reverse curls (11.3)
Erector spinae	Back of spine	Spine	Extension of the spine – straightening the spine	Back extensions (11.6)
Obliques	Side of trunk	Spine	Lateral flexion and rotation of the spine – twisting and bending the trunk to one side	Twisting sit-ups (11.2)
Pectorals	Front of the chest	Shoulder	Adduction and horizontal flexion of the arm – crossing the arms in front of the body	Press-ups (11.5) Bench press (11.31) Bent arm pullover (11.32) Lying dumbbell flyes (11.34)
Trapezius	Upper and middle back	Shoulder girdle	Extension of the neck – keeping the head up. Elevation of the shoulder – lifting and lowering the shoulders. Retraction of the scapulae – squeezing the shoulder blades together	Upright row (11.23) Prone flyes (11.35)
Latissimus dorsi	Side of the back	Shoulder	Adduction of the shoulder – drawing the arms down across the body or rowing movements of the arm	Single arm row (11.8) Bent arm pullover (11.32)
Deltoids	Top of the shoulder	Shoulder	Abduction of the shoulder – lifting the arms out to the side of the body	Dumbbell lateral raise (11.27)
Biceps	Front of the upper arm	Elbow and shoulder	Flexion of the elbow – bending the elbow	Biceps curl (11.26)

Table 10.3	Joint actions in which the major muscle groups contract concentrically, and an example of exercises to work this muscle cont.			
Triceps	Back of the upper arm	Elbow and shoulder	Extension of the elbow – straightening the elbow	Press-ups (11.5) Triceps dips (11.35 (a)) Lying triceps extension (11.55) Behind neck press (11.30) Triceps kickback (11.9)

NB: (1) this table has been adapted from *The Complete Guide to Exercise in Water*. Lawrence (A&C Black: 2004) and is designed to simplify the actions of the major muscles. More detailed and descriptive analysis of muscular work can be found in the references on page 263; (2) exercises named in the fifth column of Table 10.3 will bring about both concentric (lifting phase of the movement) and eccentric (lowering phase) muscle contractions (isotonic muscle work).

Summary for training to improve muscular strength and endurance

To improve muscular endurance, perform more repetitions of the exercise. To improve muscular strength, add further resistance to movement.

Add resistance by:
- increasing the range of motion (e.g. using a step to incline abdominal curls/sit-ups)
- decreasing the speed of the exercise (e.g. taking four counts to lift and four counts to lower)
- increasing the leverage (e.g. extending the arms over the head with arms at the side of the ears to perform an abdominal curl/sit-up)
- adding external resistance using bands, barbells, dumbbells, ankle weights, or partner work. (Stability ball exercises can be included to challenge balance and provide additional resistance for core muscles. Exercises are listed at the end of this section.)

Make the circuit harder by:
- increasing the number of stations, so that more muscles can be worked or a variety of exercises for the same muscle group can be included
- working the same muscle/muscle group more than once (multiple sets)
- increasing the number of circuits
- decreasing the rest time between stations. This will be dependent on the fitness level of the group and the intensity of the exercise being performed. Longer rest time may be needed if the exercises are strength-biased.
- super-setting specific muscle groups – e.g. a triceps exercise follows a biceps exercise, and a deltoid exercise follows a latissimus dorsi exercise
- giant setting – e.g. working the same muscle group consecutively with different exercises (press-ups, chest flyes and bench press).

NB: whether strength or endurance are improved will be dependent on the number of repetitions one is able to perform. Lower repetition ranges (1–10) will primarily improve strength. Higher repetition ranges (15–30) will primarily improve endurance. Mid-repetition ranges (10–15) will improve both to some degree, and are recommended for general muscular fitness.

MUSCULAR STRENGTH AND ENDURANCE FITNESS EXERCISES

11

NB: correct breathing is essential when performing muscular strength and endurance exercises, especially those which are more strenuous. The primary issue is that the breath is not held. Ideally, all outward breaths should occur on the effort, the lifting phase of the movement. Inward breaths should occur on the lowering phase of the exercise.

Purpose

This exercise will work the abdominal muscles at the front of the trunk (rectus abdominis).

Starting position and instructions

- Lie on your back with your knees bent and your feet firmly placed on the floor. Tighten the abdominal muscles and pull them towards the spine. Maintain this fixed position of the abdominals throughout the movement
- Place your hands either on the thighs (easier), across your chest (slightly harder), at the sides of the head (harder still), or lengthen the arms above the head (hardest).
- Contract the abdominal muscles to lift and curl the shoulders and chest upwards

Exercise 11.1	**Sit-ups/Curl-ups**

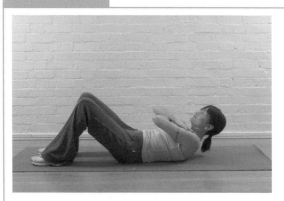

Hands across chest – can also be performed with hands on thighs, hands to side of head or hands extended at side of head

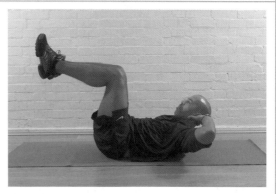

Crunch with hands to side of head – can also be performed with the hands on thighs, hands across chest or hands extended at side of head

- Lift as far as is comfortable, but without lifting the lower back off the floor
- Reverse the movement under control.

Coaching points

- Tighten the abdominal muscles
- Initiate the movement by contracting the abdominals and lifting the shoulders
- Take care not to excessively hollow or flatten the spine
- Keep the neck relaxed and look forwards, following the movement of the rest of the spine
- Control the movement upwards and downwards
- If the hands are placed at the sides of the head, support the head without 'pulling'.

Progressions/Adaptations

- Start with the shorter leverage positions explained above and progress to the longer leverage positions
- Start with a regular pace of movement and progressively decrease the speed. For example, take two counts to lift and two counts to lower.
- Perform more repetitions to increase muscular endurance
- External resistance can be placed across the chest to challenge muscular strength
- Lift the legs in the air and cross the ankles (a crunch) for variation
- A gym ball can be used to support the lower legs. This will demand greater core stability
- A full sit-up can be performed. However, this will involve working the hip flexor muscle, and great care should be taken not to allow the back to hollow and hyper-extend.

| Exercise 11.2 | Reverse curls |

Purpose

This exercise will work the muscles at the front of the trunk (rectus abdominis).

Starting position and instructions

- Lie on the back
- Lift the knees towards the chest so that they are in line with the belly button
- Keep the knees slightly bent or extend the legs, whichever is most comfortable
- Tilt the pelvis to lift the buttocks from the floor so that the knees travel closer towards the chest.

Coaching points

- Initiate the movement from the abdominals
- Pull the abdominals in tight
- Take care not to swing the legs
- Take care not to hollow the lower back when returning the movement
- Do not allow the legs to travel too far away from the central line of the body. This will place too much stress on the back.

Progressions/Adaptations

- Perform the exercise at a slower pace so that the muscles have to contract and work for longer
- As a variation, twist the legs towards the right shoulder and then the left shoulder to work the oblique muscles
- Combine the exercise with a curl-up (see Exercise 11.1) to increase motor skills and muscle work involved
- Vary the speed of the exercise, alternating slow and quick repetitions.

Exercise 11.3	Twisting sit-ups

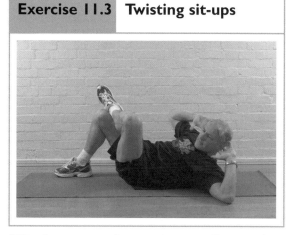

NB: the various lever positions illustrated in diagram 11.1 are equally appropriate for altering the intensity of this exercise.

Purpose

This exercise will work the abdominal muscles at the sides of the trunk (obliques). It will also work the muscles at the front of the trunk, the rectus abdominis.

Starting position and instructions

- Lie on your back with your knees bent and your feet firmly placed on the floor
- Tighten the abdominal muscles and pull them towards the spine. Maintain this fixed position of the abdominals throughout the movement
- Place your hands either on the thighs (easier), across your chest (slightly harder), at the sides of the head (harder still), or lengthen the arms above the head (hardest)
- Contract the abdominal muscles to lift and curl the shoulders and chest upwards, twisting the body to one side. Lower and repeat, twisting to the other side.

Coaching points

- Tighten the abdominal muscles
- Initiate the movement by contracting the abdominals and lifting the shoulders
- Take care not to excessively hollow or flatten the back
- Keep the neck relaxed and look forwards, following the rest of the spine
- Control the movement upwards and downwards
- If the hands are placed at the sides of the head, do not pull on the head
- Lift only as far as is comfortable, and without lifting the lower back off the floor
- Reverse the movement under control
- Ease the shoulder towards the knee rather than pulling the head over too far.

Progressions/Adaptations

- Start with the shorter leverage positions explained above and progress to the longer leverage positions
- Start with a regular pace of movement and progressively decrease the speed. For example, take two counts to lift and two counts to lower, or four counts to lift and four to lower
- Perform more repetitions to increase muscular endurance. Performing more repetitions on the same side will require greater endurance than alternating the lifts
- Lift the legs in the air and cross the ankles (a crunch) for variation
- Cycling the legs can provide further variation, but care must be taken not to twist too far or take the legs too far out. Lowering the legs too far will place unnecessary stress on the lower back
- Use a gym ball to support the legs. This demands greater core stability.

Exercise 11.4	Triceps dips

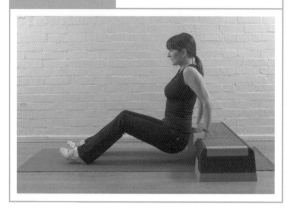

Purpose

This exercise will work the muscles at the back of the upper arms (triceps).

Starting position and instructions

- Sit on the floor with the knees bent and the feet flat on the floor
- Position the hands about 12 inches behind the buttocks, facing the body
- Bend and straighten the elbows to lift and lower the body weight
- Perform for the desired number of repetitions.

Coaching points

- Raise and lower the body under control
- Keep the abdominals pulled in tight and take care not to hollow the back
- Ensure the elbows extend fully as the body is lifted up, but do not lock the elbows
- If the buttocks are lifted off the floor, ensure the body is fixed and only the elbows move
- If the legs are extended, take care not to lock the knee joint
- On the bench, check that the elbows bend and the body lowers to a comfortable range of motion.

Progressions/Adaptations

- Triceps kickbacks without weights will be easier for less fit persons or those with a wrist injury (see Exercise 11.9)
- Start with the buttocks on the floor and progressively add resistance to the movement by (a) lifting the buttocks, (b) extending the legs and (c) performing from a bench to move through a greater range of motion
- Perform the exercise at a slower pace so that the muscles have to contract and work for longer
- Vary the speed of the exercise, combining slower and quicker movements
- Perform through different ranges of motion, i.e. halfway up and down, all the way up and halfway down, up again and all the way down, and all the way up and down
- Combine with a knee extension to add variation (ensure both legs receive equal work)
- Use a partner to press on the shoulders to add further resistance to the movement (NB: partner work needs to be conducted with great care)
- Perform with the feet and arms raised on different benches to add further resistance to the movement.

Exercise 11.5 | Press-ups

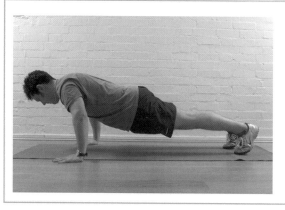 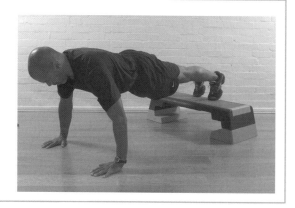

Purpose

This exercise will work the muscles at the front of the chest and shoulders (pectorals and anterior deltoid), and the muscles at the back of the upper arm (triceps).

Starting position and instructions

- Start in the position illustrated above
- Place the hands shoulder-width-and-a-half apart and level with the shoulders, fingers facing forwards
- Bend and straighten the elbows to lower and lift the body weight up and down.
- Perform the desired number of repetitions.

Coaching points

- Keep the abdominals pulled in tight and the back straight
- Keep the spine and neck in line
- Ensure the elbows fully extend but do not lock
- Keep the body weight forwards and over the shoulders to maximise the resistance
- If kneeling in the box or ¾ position, take care not to rest on the knee caps
- Ensure the body lowers and lifts in one smooth movement

- The chest should touch the floor between the shoulder blades
- Maintain a right angle (90 degrees) at the elbow joints, keeping the elbows and wrists in alignment.

Progressions/Adaptations

- The positions illustrated above show methods of adding resistance to the movement
- Perform the exercise at a slower pace so that the muscles have to contract and work for longer
- Build up to higher repetitions in each position to increase endurance. When 20 repetitions can be achieved, try a harder position
- Vary the speed of the exercise, e.g. two slow double time and four normal pace
- Combine a leg curl in-between full press-ups to add variety for stronger participants
- Adding a clap will make the movement more explosive
- As a variation, perform with the hands shoulder-width apart (narrow). Ensure the elbows move backwards rather than outwards to maintain the correct elbow and wrist alignment.

Exercise 11.6	Back extension

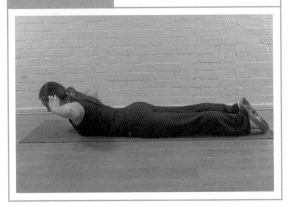

Purpose

This exercise will work the muscles that run along the length of the spine, the erector spinae.

Starting position and instructions

- Lie face down on the floor
- Place the hands either at the side of the head or on the buttocks
- Pull the abdominals in tight to fix the spine
- Raise the chest up from the floor and lower under control.

Coaching points

- Keep the neck in line with the rest of the spine
- Keep the abdominals pulled in tight and take care not to hollow the back
- Lift to a comfortable height
- Control the movement and breathe comfortably throughout.

Progressions/Adaptations

- To make the exercise easier, perform with the hands resting on the floor in front of the body and use them to support some of the body weight. Ensure that the arms are not used to push the body up from the floor
- Progressively add resistance by placing the hands on (a) the buttocks, (b) at the side of the head and (c) extending the arms (Superman) in line with the rest of the spine
- Perform the exercise at a slower pace so that the muscle has to contract for a longer period of time
- Combine with prone flyes (Exercise 11.7) to add variety for persons with greater motor skills
- Add a small rotation at the top of the lift to alternate right and left sides. Care must be taken to keep this movement under control and execute with safe and effective technique.

Exercise 11.7	**Prone flyes**

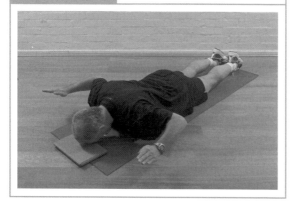

Purpose

This exercise will work the muscles in the middle of the back, the trapezius.

Starting position and instructions

- Lie or kneel in the positions illustrated above
- Keep the elbows bent and out to the side of the body, level with the shoulders
- Raise the arms from the floor using the muscles in the middle of the back. Lower them back to the floor under control

Coaching points

- Raise the arms under control
- Keep the abdominals pulled in tight and take care not to hollow the back
- Keep the elbows slightly bent
- Initiate the movement from the middle of the back
- Take care not to let the arms dictate the movement – use the arms as resistance
- If kneeling on one leg, take care not to rest on the kneecap and ensure the chest is able to rest comfortably on the thigh

- If lying, keep the hip bones pressed towards the floor and lift the belly button towards the spine.

Progressions/Adaptations

- To make the exercise easier, start with the hands on the floor at the sides of the buttocks and gently lift the shoulders up from the floor, squeezing the shoulder blades together
- Perform the exercise at a slower pace so that the muscles have to contract and work for longer
- Vary the speed of the exercise, e.g. two slow double time and four normal pace
- Progress by extending the leverage: (a) arms out to the side and the elbows bent, or (b) arms out to the side and the arms extended (keep a slight bend in the elbows)
- Add weights to make the exercise harder
- Combine with back extensions for variety
- Perform kneeling to increase the range of motion
- Perform from a step to increase the range of motion.

Exercise 11.8	Single-arm rowing

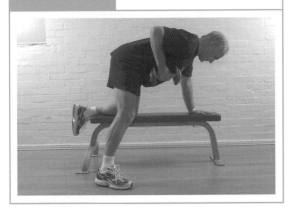

Purpose

This exercise will work the muscles at the back, the latissimus dorsi, and the muscles at the front of the upper arm, the biceps.

Starting position and instructions

- Position the dumbbell at the side of the bench
- Place one knee and one hand on the bench with the other foot level with the knee and forming a triangular base of support
- Keep the weight-bearing knee slightly bent
- Bend the knee further and extend the arm to reach for the dumbbell
- Straighten the leg to lift the dumbbell into position
- Draw the dumbbell towards the armpit, keeping the dumbbell close to the body
- Lower the dumbbell back down so that the arm is extended
- Repeat for the desired number of repetitions
- Perform using the other arm.

Coaching points

- Keep the back straight and look forwards throughout the movement
- Keep the abdominals pulled in tight
- Ensure the elbow does not lock as the dumbbell lowers back down
- Take care not to twist the back or shoulders
- Keep the shoulders square.

Progressions/Adaptations

- Perform without the weight to rehearse the movement
- Perform the exercise at a slower pace
- Vary the pace, for example two slow double time lifts and four normal pace lifts
- Combine with 'triceps kickbacks' (see Exercise 11.9) to add variety for persons with greater motor skills
- Use resistance bands.

Exercise 11.9	Triceps kickbacks

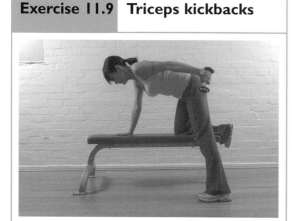

Purpose

This exercise will work the muscles at the back of the upper arm, the triceps.

Starting position and instructions

- Position the dumbbell at the side of the bench
- Place one knee and one hand on the bench with the other foot level with the knee and forming a triangular base of support
- Keep the weight-bearing knee slightly bent
- Bend the knee further and extend the arm to reach for the dumbbell
- Straighten the leg to lift the dumbbell into position
- Draw the dumbbell upwards so that the upper arm is pressed into the side of the body. Hold this position.
- Extend the elbow backwards, keeping the upper arm fixed and the dumbbell close to the body
- Return by bringing the dumbbell back to the initial held position
- Repeat for the desired number of repetitions
- Perform using the other arm.

Coaching points

- Move the dumbbell under control and do not allow the weight to swing
- Keep the abdominals pulled in tight and take care not to twist or hollow the back
- Extend the elbow fully without locking or hyper-extending the joint
- Keep the shoulders square throughout the movement.

Progressions/Adaptations

- Perform the exercise with no weight or a lighter weight to rehearse the technique
- Perform at a slower pace so that the muscles have to contract and work for longer
- Vary the speed of the exercise (combine slow time and normal time repetitions)
- Combine with single arm row (see Exercise 11.8) to add variety
- Use resistance bands instead of weights.

Exercise 11.10	The plank

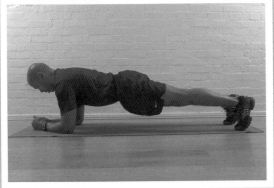

NB: this photo shows the hardest version of 'the plank', Level 3.

Purpose

This exercise will work the muscles responsible for maintaining core stability of the pelvic region, the transversus abdominis and pelvic floor muscles.

Starting position and instructions

Level 1
- Lie face down on the floor, keeping the pubic and pelvic bones level and in contact with the floor. Rest the forehead on the back of the hands
- Take a breath in
- Breathe out, pulling in the belly button (umbilicus) towards the spine and at the same time drawing up the pelvic floor muscles between the legs (imagine you are trying to stop the flow of urine)
- Hold this fixed abdominal position for between five and 10 secs, breathing normally
- Release and repeat.

Coaching points

- Ensure a neutral pelvic alignment is maintained throughout.

Progressions/Adaptations

Level 2
- A progression of this is to raise the body onto the front of the thighs and elbows (placed at the sides of the rib cage) but only once the abdominals are in a fixed position. Breathe as above

Level 3
- A further progression is to raise the body onto the elbows and toes but only once the fixed abdominal position is achieved. The body should be held in a straight position with the shoulders relaxed and away from the ears (not hunched). Breathe as above and ensure the abdominals remain contracted.

Exercise 11.11	Side bends with weights/bands

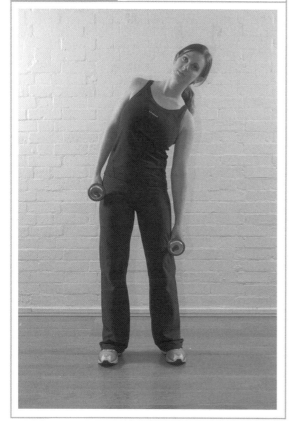

Purpose

This exercise will strengthen the oblique muscles at the sides of the trunk.

Starting position and instructions

- Start with the feet hip-width apart, the body upright and the knees unlocked
- Hold a weight in each hand or use a band
- Bend directly to the right side in a controlled manner
- Return to the central position
- Bend directly to the left side in a controlled manner
- Return to the central position
- Perform for the desired number of repetitions.

Coaching points

- Bend only as far over as is comfortable
- Keep the hips facing forwards and avoid hollowing of the lower back by tightening the abdominal muscles
- Keep the movement controlled
- Keep the body lifted between the hips and the ribs
- Lift up before bending to the side
- Lean directly to the side and ensure the body does not roll forwards or backwards
- Visualise your body as being placed between two panes of glass.

Progressions/Adaptations

- Start without weights to develop the technique
- Start with a smaller bend and progress to a slightly larger range of motion, but only as far as is comfortable
- Start by alternating the bending movement from right to left and progress by performing more repetitions to one side before changing sides. This will require slightly greater muscular endurance to maintain correct alignment
- Increase the resistance lifted by using heavier dumbbells or a stronger resistance band.

Exercise 11.12	Seated row

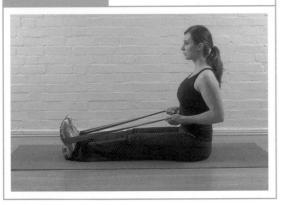

Purpose

This exercise will strengthen the muscles at the front of the upper arm and at the side of the back (biceps and latissimus dorsi).

Starting position and instructions

- Take up a seated position on a mat with legs straight and a slight bend in the knee
- Wrap a rubber resistance band around the feet, holding on to each end with the hands
- Leading with the elbow and keeping the arms close to the body, pull the hands back towards the body. Return to extended arm position and repeat.

Coaching points

- Keep the chest lifted, the back straight and the knees unlocked
- The elbows lead the movement and remain close to the body
- Sit up straight with the back in an upright position
- Maintain a strong, firm wrist position throughout.

Progressions/Adaptations

- Use a lighter strength band initially and progress to using a stronger band
- Perform on fixed resistance weight training equipment
- Perform with a squeeze of the shoulder blades to work the trapezius.

Exercise 11.13	Pec dec

Purpose

This exercise will strengthen the pectoral muscles at the front of the chest.

Starting position and instructions

- Lie on a mat with knees bent and feet flat on the floor
- Place the arms to the sides of the body, level with the shoulders, and bend the elbows to a right-angle position
- Keeping the elbows fixed in this position, lift the arms until they meet together over the chest, then return them to the floor
- Repeat.

Coaching points

- Keep the abdominals tight to stabilise the spine
- Control the movement of the arms.

Progressions/Adaptations

- To increase the intensity, dumbbells can be held in the hands
- Perform on fixed-resistance weight-training equipment
- Perform seated with an exercise band behind the back or attached to a wall bar.

Exercise 11.14	Straight-arm pull

Purpose

This exercise will strengthen the muscles at the sides of the back (latissimus dorsi).

Starting position and instructions

- Adopt an upright position facing wall bars or similar anchor points
- Attach two resistance bands approximately twice shoulder-width apart at a height enabling the participant to reach them at just above head level
- Stand with feet shoulder-width apart, soft knees and leaning slightly forwards
- Grasp the ends of the resistance bands and, keeping the arms straight with a slight bend in the elbows, draw the arms inwards and down towards the thighs
- Return to the start position
- Repeat.

Coaching points

- Control the movement
- Keep the abdominals fixed and the back straight.

Progressions/Adaptations

- Start with a lighter resistance band and progressively use a stronger band
- Perform using fixed-resistance equipment.

Exercise 11.15	Triceps press/ extension

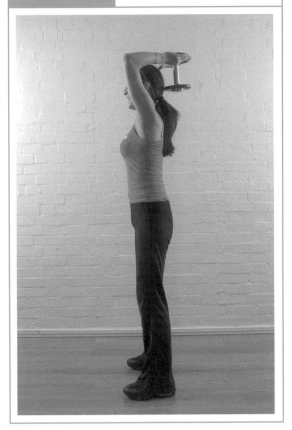

Coaching points

- Ensure a slight bend is maintained at the elbow when full extension is achieved
- Keep the abdominals tight and the chest lifted
- If standing, bend the knees slightly and adopt a shoulder-width foot stance
- Look forwards.

Progressions/Adaptations

- Start without a weight
- Progressively lift heavier weights
- Perform with an exercise band by holding one end of the band in each hand (behind the back). Keeping the lower arm still, only move the top arm – extend before lowering.

Purpose

This exercise will strengthen the muscles at the back of the upper arms (triceps).

Starting position and instructions

- Adopt either a seated or standing position
- Use either a resistance band or dumbbell held above the head
- Bending at the elbow, lower the resistance down
- When full flexion has been achieved, return the resistance back to the start position above the head.

Exercise 11.16	Hamstring curls

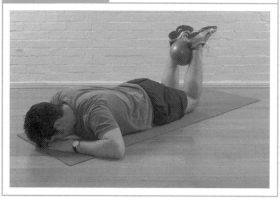

Purpose

This exercise will strengthen the muscles at the back of the thighs (hamstrings).

Starting position and instructions

- Lie face down on a mat
- Place a dumbbell between the feet
- Bend the knees and curl the weight towards the bottom while keeping the upper legs in contact with the floor.

Coaching points

- Maintain a fixed abdominal posture
- Control the movements and don't lock the knees
- Keep the upper legs in contact with the floor.

Progressions/Adaptations

- Start without a weight and progressively increase the resistance lifted
- Perform in the standing position using a resistance band anchored to the opposite leg.

Exercise 11.17	Shoulder shrugs

Purpose

This exercise will strengthen the muscles of the upper back (trapezius).

Starting position and instructions

- Stand with feet shoulder-width apart
- Hold on to either dumbbells or resistance bands (secured under the feet)
- Keep the arms straight and raise/shrug the shoulders up towards the ears slowly and lower under control
- Repeat.

Coaching points

- Maintain an upright posture
- Keep the abdominals tight, the spine upright and the chin parallel to the floor
- Keep the knees unlocked and the chest lifted
- Control the movements.

Progressions/Adaptations

- Start without a weight
- Lift progressively heavier weights.

Exercise 11.18	Bent forward rowing

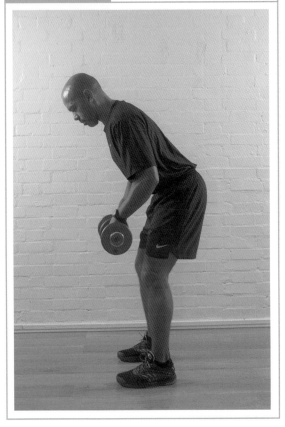

Purpose

This exercise will strengthen the muscles at the sides of the back and front of the upper arms, the latissimus dorsi and biceps.

Starting position and instructions

- Stand with feet hip-width apart and knees bent
- Take hold of a pair of dumbbells and lean forwards slightly at the hip (no more than 45 degrees)
- Start with the arms fully extended (straight) with just a slight bend in the elbows

- Pull the arms towards the chest, leading with the elbows
- Lower under control and repeat.

Coaching points

- Keep the chest lifted and look forwards
- Keep the head and spine in line
- Maintain good core stability by pulling in the abdominals
- Keep the wrists fixed throughout.

Progressions/Adaptations

- Start without weights and lift progressively heavier weights
- As an adaptation, perform a single arm row with one hand supported on the thigh (one arm at a time).

Exercise 11.19	Sand lizard

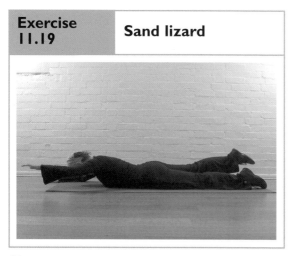

- Progress to performing the combined arm and leg action
- Very small weights can be added but take care as this may place undue stress on the back.

Purpose

This exercise will strengthen the buttock muscles (gluteals) and the muscles between the shoulder blades (rhomboids and trapezius).

Starting position and instructions

- Lie face down with the arms extended over the head in front of the body
- Raise one leg off the floor and at the same time raise the opposite arm off the floor
- Repeat with the other arm and leg.

Coaching points

- Keep the neck in line with the rest of the spine
- Keep the abdominals pulled in tight and take care not to hollow the back
- Lift to a comfortable height
- Control the movement and breathe comfortably throughout.

Progressions/Adaptations

- Start by performing the arm action and leg action in isolation

Exercise 11.20	Rotator cuff

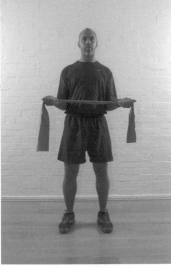

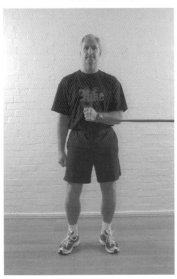

Starting position and instructions

External rotation

- Adopt an upright body position and maintain core stability of the pelvis
- Take hold of a resistance band, one end in each hand
- Keep a right angle at each elbow joint and the upper arm locked into the side of the body at the start of the movement
- Turn (rotate) both arms outwards from the shoulder joints, pulling the resistance band outwards. Slowly return to the start position.

Internal rotation

- Secure the resistance band to the wall or similar (if comfortable, hold the band in each hand behind the back, keeping the elbows in to the sides)
- Start with the arm fully rotated outwards, take hold of the resistance band, then pull the arm inwards. Maintain a fixed elbow position and rotate the arm towards the centre line of the body
- Repeat with the other arm.

Coaching points

- Keep a right angle at each elbow joint and the upper arm locked into the side of the body throughout the movement
- Maintain an upright posture
- Make sure the knees are unlocked.

Progressions/Adaptations

- Start without a resistance band
- Use progressively stronger resistance bands to intensify the movement.

Purpose

This exercise will strengthen the internal and external rotator cuff muscles (teres major and minor, infraspinatus, supraspinatus and subscapulans).

Exercise 11.21	The dead-lift

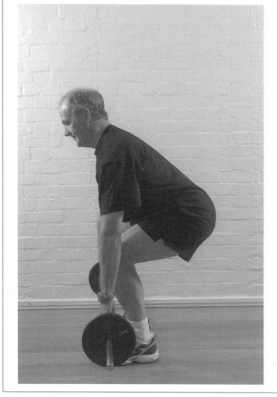

NB: this exercise should be used whenever a weight or object needs to be lifted to the thighs. It allows the weight to be carried by the stronger thigh muscles and therefore prevents injury to the back if lifting incorrectly.

Purpose

This exercise will work the buttock muscles (gluteus maximus), back muscles (erector spinae) and the muscles at the front of the thigh (quadriceps).

Starting position and instructions

- Place the toes underneath the barbell, approximately hip-width apart

- Ensure the body is positioned central to the barbell
- Bend at the knees and hips and take an overhand grip of the bar
- Lift the bar from the floor by straightening the knees and hips and leading the movement with the shoulders.

Coaching points

- Ensure that the back is straight and abdominals pulled in
- Take care not to hollow the back
- Push the buttocks backwards and don't let the knees travel too far forwards of the bar
- The bottom should be higher than the knees when bending to reach the bar
- Look forwards and slightly upwards
- Keep the bar close to the body throughout the movement
- Ensure the body moves to a fully extended position without locking the joints (hip and knee fully straightened and spine extended).

Progressions/Adaptations

- Perform the exercise without a barbell to get used to the position
- Start by lifting a lighter weight and progress to a heavier weight
- Start at a slower pace so that the muscles have to contract and work for longer
- Vary the speed of the movements, for example some very slow (four counts down and four counts up) and some to normal time
- Combine with a calf raise to add variety to the movement
- Combine with an upright row to add variety to the movement.

NB: the last two variations provide a method for breaking down and introducing another lift 'clean' into the session.

Exercise 11.22	Upright row

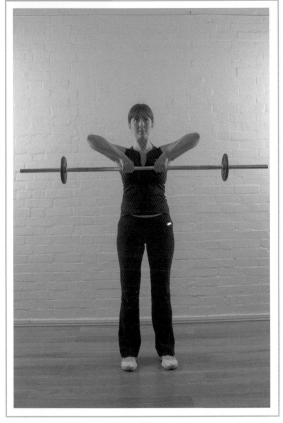

Purpose

This exercise will work the muscles at the front of the shoulders (anterior deltoid), the front of the upper arms (biceps and brachialis), and the top of the back (trapezius).

Starting position and instructions

- Dead-lift the barbell to the thighs using an overhand grip
- Widen the foot stance to hip-width and a half apart
- Narrow the bar grip to double-thumb-width apart

- Keep a firm grip of the bar with the thumbs tucked under
- Raise the bar towards the chin, keeping the bar close to the body
- Lower the bar under control
- Repeat for the desired number of repetitions.

Coaching points

- Keep the bar close to the body
- Keep the abdominals pulled in tight and avoid hollowing the lower back on the downward phase
- Keep the movement controlled
- Tuck the bottom under and keep the knees unlocked
- Lead the movement with the elbows, lifting them as high as possible (up to the chin).

Progressions/Adaptations

- Perform without a weight to rehearse the movement
- Perform with a lighter barbell and progressively add resistance
- Perform at a slower pace so that the muscles have to contract and work for longer
- Combine with a dead-lift to perform part of 'the clean'.

N.B. A wider grip can be adopted for those people with low levels of shoulder mobility and/or rotator cuff problems. The bar can also be lifted to a lower height.

Exercise 11.23	Calf raise

Purpose

This exercise will work the muscles at the back of the lower leg, the gastrocnemius and soleus.

Starting position and instructions

- Stand with the feet hip-width apart
- Dead-lift the barbell to the thighs using an overhand grip
- Keep the bar still
- Rise on to the balls of the feet, lifting the heels from the floor
- Lower down under control
- Perform for the desired number of repetitions.

Coaching points

- Keep the bar still and close to the body
- Keep the abdominals pulled in tight and the back straight
- Keep the knee joints unlocked
- Press onto the balls of the feet with the weight central; take care not to roll the ankles outwards
- Keep the movement smooth and controlled.

Progressions/Adaptations

- Perform without a weight to rehearse the movement
- Perform with a lighter barbell and progressively add resistance
- Perform at a slower pace so that the muscles have to contract and work for longer
- Combine with a dead-lift to perform part of 'the clean'
- Perform with an upright row to increase motor skills and rehearse as part of the clean

- Perform with a bent knee to isolate the soleus muscle.

Exercise 11.24	Toe tapping and wrist curls

Purpose

This exercise will strengthen the muscles at the front of the shins (tibialis anterior) and the forearms (wrist flexor and extensor muscles).

Starting position and instructions

- Stand with the feet hip-width apart, maintaining a slight bend in the knees
- Lift the toes alternately off the floor as high as possible (dorsiflexion)
- At the same time, hold on to a small bar with a rope tied to it. At the other end of the rope, tie a weight. Roll the bar around using a wringing action of the wrist
- Reverse the action to lower the weight to the floor.

Coaching points

- Keep the elbows in to the sides of the body
- Maintain a right angle at the elbow joint
- Roll the bar around under control using the wrist to wind the rope/weight up to touch the bar
- Maintain an upright posture.

Progressions/Adaptations

- Start without a weight and progressively increase the weight
- Start with a shorter rope and progressively lengthen the rope/band
- Start slowly and move progressively faster.

Exercise 11.25	Dumbbell lunge

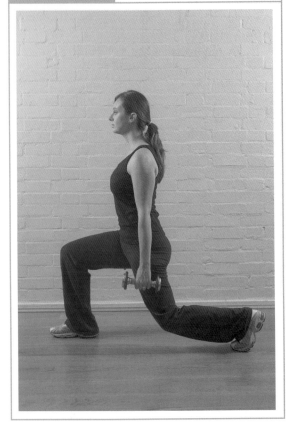

Purpose

This exercise will work the buttock muscles (gluteus maximus) and the muscles at the front of the thighs (quadriceps).

Starting position and instructions

- Stand with the feet hip-width apart with dumbbells placed each side of the feet
- Dead-lift the dumbbells to the thighs
- Check that the feet are positioned comfortably at hip-width apart, toes facing forwards
- Take a large step forwards and bend the knee to lower the body weight downwards
- Ensure both knees are positioned at right angles (90 degrees)

- Push through the thigh to lift the body back to an extended position
- Perform either by alternating legs or repeating the movement on the same leg
- Dead-lift the dumbbells to the floor on completion of the exercise.

Coaching points

- Ensure the front knee does not overshoot the toe
- Step forwards and sink the body down rather than diving forwards into the movement
- Keep the abdominals pulled in tight and the chest lifted
- Ensure the knee does not roll inwards
- Bend the back knee towards the floor but ensure the kneecap does not crash against the floor
- Look straight ahead and slightly down
- Drive through the thigh to return the body to an upright position
- Keep a relaxed grip on the dumbbells and keep the shoulders relaxed and pressed down.

Progressions/Adaptations

- Perform without a weight to rehearse the movement and to familiarise participants with the balance required
- Perform through a smaller range of motion initially
- Start the exercise at a slower pace so that the muscles have to contract and work for longer
- Start with lighter dumbbells and progressively add weight
- Vary the speed of the exercise, for example two slow double time and four normal pace
- Alternating legs will be slightly easier; performing a number of repetitions on the same leg will require greater muscular endurance

- Perform with one leg raised backwards and resting on a box/step. All repetitions are performed by the supporting leg, requiring greater muscular endurance and balance
- Can be performed travelling forwards.

Exercise 11.26	Biceps curl

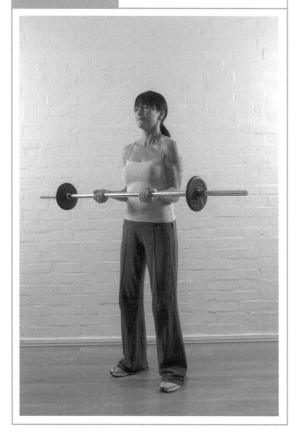

Purpose
This exercise will work the muscles at the front of the upper arms (biceps and brachialis).

Starting position and instructions
- Stand with the feet hip-width apart
- Dead-lift the barbell to the thighs using an underhand grip
- Widen the foot stance to shoulder-width-and-a-half apart and unlock the knees
- Narrow the grip of the barbell to shoulder-width apart
- Fix the elbows in to the sides of the body
- Keep the body lifted and the buttocks tucked under
- Curl the bar in an arc-like motion towards the chest
- Lower the bar to the thighs and fully extend (not locking) the elbow.

Coaching points
- Raise the bar under control
- Keep the abdominals pulled in tight and take care not to hollow or swing the back
- Keep the wrists fixed and straight
- Keep the elbows and upper arms close to the body
- The lower arms should be the only body parts moving
- Avoid locking the elbows when the bar lowers but reach a full extension.

Progressions/Adaptations
- Perform without a bar (or a light bar) to rehearse the skill
- Progressively add greater weight to the movement
- Perform at a slower pace so that the muscles have to contract and work for longer
- Vary the speed of the exercise, for example two slow double time and four normal pace
- Perform through different ranges of motion, i.e. halfway up and down, all the way up and halfway down, up again and all the way down, and all the way up and down
- Perform with dumbbells or resistance bands to add variety
- Perform with a rotation using dumbbells.

Exercise 11.27	Dumbbell lateral/frontal raises

Purpose

This exercise will work the shoulder muscles. The lateral raise works the medial deltoid and the frontal raise works the anterior deltoid.

Starting position and instructions

- Stand with the feet hip-width apart
- Dead-lift the dumbbells to the thighs
- Widen the foot stance to hip-width-and-a-half apart
- Position the dumbbells at the sides of the thighs
- Raise the dumbbells out to the sides of the body at shoulder height
- Lower the dumbbells under control.

Coaching points

- Lead the movement with the knuckles and keep the wrists fixed
- Keep the elbows slightly bent throughout the movement
- Keep the abdominals pulled in tight and the bottom tucked under
- Rotate the dumbbells as they are lifted so that the thumbs tilt forwards
- Avoid any excess movement at the top of the back
- Keep the movement controlled and smooth.

Progressions/Adaptations

- Perform without the weights to rehearse the movement
- Perform the exercise at a slower pace so that the muscles have to contract and work for longer
- Vary the speed of the exercise, for example use some slow time and some normal time
- Combine with a dumbbell lunge to challenge motor skills
- Raise the dumbbells to the front to emphasise work on the anterior deltoid.

Exercise 11.28	The clean

NB: this is an extremely complex lift. It is explained in this text purely to show readers an appropriate method for lifting a weight or object over the head. It will need to be performed to move the barbell into position for the back squat and behind neck press. It is not intended to be performed as a specific exercise.

Safety note: this exercise needs to be supervised and instructed by a qualified resistance training teacher. It should not be performed unsupervised by persons inexperienced at working with weights.

Purpose

This exercise works many of the major muscles. The buttock muscles (gluteus maximus), the back muscles (erector spinae), the muscles at the front of the thigh (quadriceps), the calf muscles (gastrocnemius and soleus), the shoulder muscles (the deltoid), the middle and upper back muscles (trapezius) and the muscles at the front of the upper arm (biceps).

Starting position/instructions/coaching points

Part 1

- Dead-lift the bar to the thighs (refer to coaching points for the dead-lift on p. 139).

Part 2

- Upright row the bar and calf raise (refer to coaching points for the upright row on p. 140 and calf raise on p. 141)

Part 3 – Receive

- Bring the elbows forwards and under the bar so that the bar rests under the shoulders. At the same time, lower the heels and bend the knees to cushion the weight
- Stand up straight; coaching point – the bar should remain in the same position.

Part 4 – Return

- Bring the elbows back around to the upright row position; coaching point – keep the bar close to the body and the elbows high
- Lower the bar to the thighs

Part 5

- Reverse dead-lift the bar to the floor (see coaching points for the dead-lift on p. 139).

Coaching points

- Keep the back straight.
- Keep the abdominals pulled in throughout the movement.

Progressions/Adaptations

- Perform the exercise without a barbell to get used to the movement.
- Perform the exercise slowly and in separate stages to get used to each phase. Aim to perform a smooth and fluid movement.

Exercise 11.29	Back squat

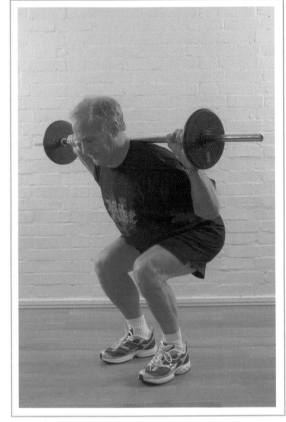

NB: see note for 'the clean' on p. 144–5 (Exercise 11.28).

Purpose

This exercise will work the buttock muscles (gluteus maximus) and the muscles at the front of the thighs (quadriceps).

Starting position and instructions

- Clean the barbell to the receive position
- Push press the bar over the head to rest at the back of the shoulders (bend the knees and push through the thighs to assist movement of the bar)
- Widen the bar grip to a comfortable position
- Ensure the feet are placed at hip-width apart
- Bend the knees and lower the body downwards
- Return to an upright position to complete the lift
- Perform for the desired number of repetitions
- To return the bar, push press the bar back over the head to rest at the front of the chest/shoulders and return as for the clean.

Coaching points

- Look forwards throughout the movement
- Keep the knees travelling in line with the feet
- Do not let the bottom drop below the knees when squatting downwards. This would place a lot of stress on the knee joints
- Keep the back straight
- Squat down so that the bar moves in a straight and vertical line
- When straightening do not lock the knees
- Fully extend the hips and knees.

Progressions/Adaptations

- Perform without the weight to rehearse the movement
- Perform at a slower pace so that the muscles have to contract and work for longer
- Perform through a smaller range of motion initially
- Progressively add weight to the barbell to increase resistance.

Exercise 11.30	Behind neck press/shoulder press

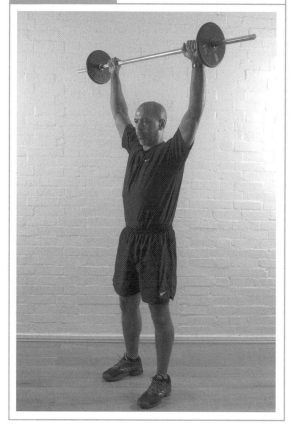

Purpose

This exercise will work the shoulder muscles (deltoids), the muscles of the upper back (trapezius) and the muscles at the back of the upper arms (triceps).

Starting position and instructions

- Clean the bar to the receive position
- Push press the bar over the head to rest at the back of the shoulders
- Widen the foot stance to hip-width-and-a-half apart to assist balance
- Widen the grip of the bar to shoulder-width-and-a-half apart

- Press the bar upwards
- Lower the bar down under control. Repeat for the desired number of repetitions
- Do not allow the bar to rest on the shoulders in-between lifts; keep a constant muscle tension
- To return the bar, narrow the grip, push the bar over the head to rest on the front of the chest/shoulders and return as for the clean.

Coaching points

- Keep the back straight, abdominals pulled in and bottom tucked under
- Keep the knuckles facing up and the wrists fixed
- Take care not to hollow the back or lock the elbows
- Keep the knees slightly bent throughout the movement
- Perform a smooth and comfortable movement.

Progressions/Adaptations

- Perform without the weight to rehearse the movement
- Add weight progressively to challenge the muscles
- Perform the exercise at a slower pace so that the muscles have to contract and work for longer
- Vary the speed of the exercise. Combine some slow reps and some faster reps
- Perform the exercise seated to protect the lumbar spine when lifting heavier weights
- Vary the exercise further by using dumbbells or resistance bands. The arms can then be pressed either together or alternately
- Stagger foot stance to assist balance (one forwards, one backwards)
- Press bar from front.

Safety Note
An alternate foot stance is to position one foot forward and one foot back. For those with low shoulder flexibility, this press can be performed to the front.

Bench lifts

In a weight-training environment all bench-based lifts should be performed using a spotter, especially for persons less experienced at lifting weights, and when heavier weights are being used.

As the focus of this book is circuit training, it is therefore assumed that the weights being lifted will not be maximal and also that weights will only be introduced to those who have some experience of training. An appropriate method of moving the bar into position for bench lifts used within a circuit training session is outlined in Table 11.1.

Table 11.1 Positioning the bar for bench lifts		
If using lighter weights and the bench lifts are performed by persons of a reasonable level of experience, it is appropriate to roll the barbell or dumbbells into position. This can be achieved in the following ways:		
Barbell	• Sit down on the bench. Lean forwards, abdominals tight, and dead-lift the bar so it rests on the thighs • Lie back flat on the bench and roll the bar over the body towards the chest. Take the appropriate grip of the bar and perform the lift • Return the bar using the same principles (roll back, sit up, stand up and return dead-lift)	
Dumbbells	• Sit down on the bench. Lean forwards, abdominals tight, and dead-lift the bar so it rests on the thighs • Lie back flat on the bench and lift alternate dumbbells to the chest • Return the dumbbells using the same principles (place back, sit up, stand up and return dead-lift)	

Exercise 11.31	Bench press (flat or inclined)

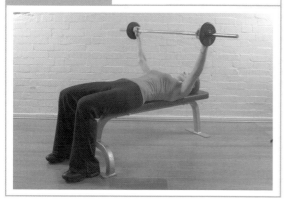

NB: if the back hollows, place a step at each side of the bench on which to rest the feet. This provides better balance and is therefore generally more secure and safer than placing the feet onto the bench.

Purpose

This exercise will work the muscles at the front of the chest (pectorals), the muscles at the front of the shoulder (anterior deltoids) and the muscles at the back of the upper arms (triceps).

Starting position and instructions

- Get the bar into position using the technique explained in Table 11.1
- Grip the bar with hands shoulder-width-and-a-half apart
- Push the bar straight up to the ceiling
- Lower the bar back to the chest under control
- Perform the desired number of repetitions
- To return the bar, follow the instructions outlined in Table 11.1.

Coaching points

- Keep the knuckles facing upwards and the wrists fixed
- Keep the abdominals pulled in tight and take care not to hollow the back (see note above)
- Move the bar in a straight line level with the chest
- Extend the arms fully but do not lock the elbows
- Keep the elbows and wrists in line and vertical as the bar lowers
- Keep the movement smooth and under control.

Progressions/Adaptations

- Perform without the weight to rehearse the movement
- Perform the exercise at a slower pace so that the muscles have to contract and work for longer
- Vary the speed of the exercise, for example performing some repetitions at slow time and some at normal pace
- Perform through different ranges of motion (lower range; upper range; full range)
- Add greater resistance to the movement by lifting a progressively heavier weight
- Use dumbbells to achieve a fuller range of motion.

Exercise 11.32	Bent arm pullover

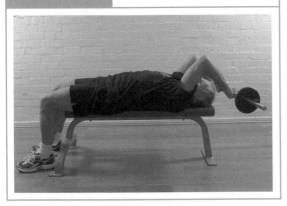

NB: if the back hollows, place a step at each side of the bench on which to rest the feet. This provides better balance and is therefore generally more secure and safer than placing the feet onto the bench.

Purpose

This exercise will work the muscles at the front of the chest, the pectorals, and the muscles at the sides of the back, the latissimus dorsi.

Starting position and instructions

- Get the bar into position using the technique explained in Table 11.1
- Take a shoulder-width grip of the bar
- Press the bar to the ceiling and lower down so that the elbows are pressed into the sides and the wrists (and bar) are in line with the elbows. Keep this 90-degree angle at the elbow throughout the movement
- Take the bar over the head, keeping the elbows fixed and in, and lower the bar towards the floor at the back of the bench
- Return by reversing the movement and leading with the elbows to bring the bar back in towards the chest

- Perform the desired number of repetitions
- To return the bar, follow the instructions outlined in Table 11.1.

Coaching points

- Move the bar under control
- Keep the abdominals pulled in tight and take care not to hollow the back, especially as the bar moves over the head and towards the floor
- Keep the elbows bent and pressed inwards (not splaying out) throughout the movement
- Breathe in a controlled manner throughout the exercise.

Progressions/Adaptations

- Perform without the weight so that the correct alignment can be rehearsed
- Add weight to the movement, by lifting a progressively heavier barbell
- Perform the exercise at a slower pace so that the muscles have to contract and work for longer
- Perform with a dumbbell to increase the range of motion and vary the exercise.

Exercise 11.33	Lying triceps extension

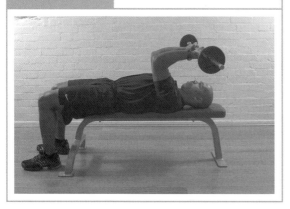

NB: if the back hollows, place a step at each side of the bench on which to rest the feet. This provides better balance and is therefore generally more secure and safer than placing the feet onto the bench.

Purpose

This exercise will work the muscles at the back of the upper arms (triceps).

Starting position and instructions

- Get the bar into position using the technique explained in Table 11.1.
- Take a shoulder-width, narrow grip of the bar
- Press the bar to the ceiling, level with the chest
- Keep the upper arms fixed in this position
- Bend the lower arms so that the barbell moves downwards towards the bridge of the nose
- Return the barbell back up to the ceiling
- Perform the desired number of repetitions
- To return the bar, follow the instructions outlined in Table 11.1.

Coaching points

- Keep the wrists and elbows fixed throughout the movement
- Keep the abdominals pulled in tight and take care not to hollow the back
- Move the bar under control
- Straighten the arms fully but without locking the elbows.

Progressions/Adaptations

- Perform the exercise without weights to rehearse the movement
- Perform the exercise at a slower pace so that the muscles have to contract and work for longer
- Vary the speed by performing some slow and extra slow counts and some normal pace counts
- For advanced and more flexible participants, take the bar down over the head. This will provide a greater range of motion and target the longer head of the triceps muscle
- Use dumbbells to work through a greater range of motion and add variety.

Exercise 11.34	Lying dumbbell flyes (flat/incline)

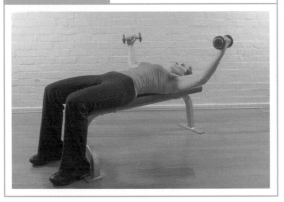

NB: if the back hollows, place a step at each side of the bench on which to rest the feet. This provides better balance and is therefore generally more secure and safer than placing the feet onto the bench.

Purpose

This exercise will work the muscles of the chest (pectorals).

Starting position and instructions

- Get the dumbbells into position by using the technique explained in Table 11.1, page 148
- Press the dumbbells to the ceiling and level with the chest, palms facing inwards
- Keep the elbows unlocked and the arms fixed in this position
- Lower the dumbbells out to each side of the body, parallel to the floor
- Return the dumbbells back in towards the body
- Perform the desired number of repetitions
- To return the dumbbells, follow the instructions outlined in Table 11.1, page 148.

Coaching points

- Move the dumbbells under control
- Keep the abdominals pulled in tight and take care not to hollow the back
- Keep the wrists, elbows and shoulders in line throughout the movement
- Keep the wrists fixed and the elbows unlocked.

Progressions/Adaptations

- Perform the exercise without the weights to rehearse the movement
- Perform at a slower pace so that the muscles have to contract and work for longer
- Vary the speed of the exercise by performing some slow double-time repetitions and some normal-pace repetitions
- Progressively add weight to increase the resistance being lifted
- This exercise can be performed on an incline or decline to focus the work on a different area of the muscle
- The exercise can also be performed with a small rotation on the downward phase so that the arms finish in a bench press position.

MSE exercises using the step or a bench to alter intensity

Upper body exercises while stepping

Light dumbbells can be used when performing stepping actions in a circuit training session. This will require additional motor skills to control dumbbells and perform stepping action safely and through a full range of motion.

Example exercises that can be performed with basic stepping actions include:
- Biceps curls

- Shoulder press
- Upright row
- Lateral arm raises
- Triceps kick-backs
- Front arm raises

Upper body exercises performed using a step or bench

Exercise 11.35 (a)	Triceps dips

Use step to increase range of motion, for example:
- Hands on the step, feet on the floor, knees bent (as shown here)
- Hands on the step, feet on the floor, legs straight
- Hands on the step and feet raised onto another step
- Increase step height.

Exercise 11.35 (b)	Press-ups

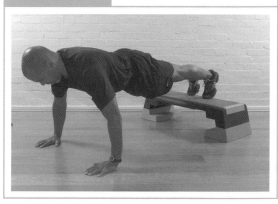

Use step to increase range of motion, for example:
- Hands on the step to decrease the range of motion
- Feet or knees on the step and hands on the floor to increase the range of motion
- Hands and feet on the step to demand greater fixation and balance
- Hands placed between two steps to demand greater core stability
- Hands and feet placed between four steps to demand greater core stability.

Exercise 11.35 (c)	Prone flyes

Use step to increase range of motion, for example:
- Lying on the step with hands at the side of the step will increase range of motion
- Add weights to increase resistance.

Trunk exercises performed using a step

Exercise 11.36 (a)	Reverse curls

Use step to increase range of motion, for example:
- Incline (head at high end of step) to increase range of motion
- Decline (head at low end of step) to decrease range of motion.

Exercise 11.36 (b)	Sit-ups/curls-ups

Use step to increase range of motion, for example:
- Incline (head at low end of step) to increase range of motion

- Decline (head at high end of step) to decrease range of motion.

Exercise 11.36 (c)	Twisting sit-ups

Use step to increase range of motion, for example:
- Incline (head at low end of step) to increase range of motion
- Decline (head at high end of step) to decrease range of motion.

Exercise 11.36 (d)	Back raise

Use step to increase range of motion, for example:
- Incline (with head at low end of step) to increase range of motion
- Decline (with head at high end of step) to decrease range of motion.

Working with core stability balls in a circuit

The core muscles of the trunk are those that surround the middle section of the body from the ribcage to the pelvis and which hold the mid-section firm to provide a strong and stable base from which other movements of the limbs can be performed safely and effectively. See Table 11.2 for information on the core muscles.

Training to strengthen the core muscles has become more of a focus in recent years and there are numerous pieces of small equipment designed to challenge core stability. One of the most popular pieces of equipment is the core stability ball (or gym ball). This section introduces exercises using the stability ball.

A key safety issue for trainers is that the core muscles need to be of a sufficient strength before progressing to using equipment. For other safety issues, see box below.

The benefits of working with stability balls

Working with a stability ball provides a challenge to existing core stability, the strength of core muscles (trunk) and balance, stabilisation and proprioception. Progressing to working with a stability ball can assist with:
- improvement of the appearance of the abdominal region (flatter abdominal area)
- reduction of low back pain and back problems
- improvement of posture and alignment
- improvement of functional movement patterns.

General safety considerations when working with core stability balls in a circuit

- Progress exercises steadily according to individual needs
- Make sure the balls are inflated to the correct height for the users (not over-inflated)
- Place on a stable surface with no sharp objects on the floor
- Ensure the balls are secure during the circuit and unable to roll and obstruct other circuit exercises
- Store the balls away from direct heat or sunlight that may cause heat distortion
- Clean regularly
- Use a rack for storage
- Inflate new balls to two-thirds of full capacity and leave for 24 hours before inflating fully
- Allow a space around the ball to exercise safely
- Check manufacturer's guidelines to find out how much weight the ball can withstand. Most balls can hold up to 300kg.

Table 11.2	The core muscles	
Muscle name	**Position**	**Function**
Front of abdominal wall (anterior)		
Rectus abdominis	Front abdomen. Runs vertically from lower ribs to pubic bone	Flexion of the spine
Transverses abdominus	Runs horizontally around the abdomen from the pelvis and the spinal extensors to the rectus abdominis	Supports the spine and pulls in the abdominals during coughing, laughing, sneezing
Side of abdominal wall (lateral)		
Internal and external obliques	Side of trunk. Run diagonally from pelvis to ribs	Internal – stabilise the spine External – rotate and laterally flex the spine
Quadratus lumborum	Side and back of the trunk. Runs from the ribcage to the pelvis	Stabilises the spine when an external force tries to bend the spine sideways (eg. carrying a suitcase)
Back of abdominal wall (posterior)		
Multifidus	A deeper muscle. Attaching to the transverses muscle and the spinous processes	Extension of individual sections of the spine.
Erector spinae	Runs down the back of the spine. Attaching from the base of the skull to the sacrum (base of the spine), pelvis and thorax	Extension of the spine and rotation of the thoracic spine.
Pelvic floor		
Pelvic floor	Positioned like a hammock underneath the pelvis. Runs from pubic bone to coccyx	Works with other abdominal muscles.

Exercise 11.37	Bridge – floor-lying with feet on ball

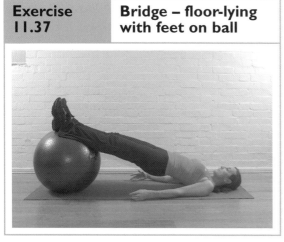

Purpose

To strengthen the muscles that keep the pelvis firm and stable.

Starting position and instructions

- Lie on your back with knees slightly bent and feet shoulder-width apart on the ball
- Find the neutral pelvic position and maintain this throughout
- Relax the shoulders, arms by the side, and lengthen the spine.

Coaching Points

- Pull the tummy in and lightly press back down into floor
- Squeeze the buttock muscles tight and curl the spine one vertebra at a time to lift the hips from the floor, aiming for hips level and in line with armpits
- Make sure the back doesn't hollow and the body weight doesn't rise up to the neck
- Breathe normally throughout the movement
- Hold for 10 secs at the top of the movement, breathing normally
- Control the upward and downward phases of the movement

- Keep the abdominals in tight throughout
- Allow the buttock-squeeze to initiate and maintain control of the movement.

Progression

- Straighten the knee on one leg, taking the weight onto the other leg (keep the pelvis firm).

Exercise 11.38	Bridge and roll – floor-lying with feet on ball

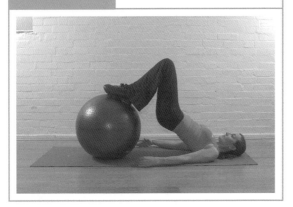

Purpose

To strengthen the muscles that keep the pelvis firm and stable, and to strengthen the back of the thigh (hamstrings).

Starting position and instructions

- Roll up into bridge position (see exercise description for bridge)
- Position feet on ball and roll ball towards buttocks
- Straighten legs and roll ball away from buttocks under control.

Coaching Points

- From bridge start position, pull the tummy in and maintain contraction of the gluteals
- Keep the abdominals in tight throughout
- Take care not to lock the knees.

Progression

- Single leg roll as progression.

Exercise 11.39	Sit-ups/Curl-ups (with and without a twist) – floor-lying with feet on ball

Purpose

This exercise will work the abdominal muscles at the front of the trunk (rectus abdominis).

Starting position and instructions

- Lying on floor, position feet in centre of ball at hip-width, with knees bent
- Maintain neutral pelvis
- Hollow the abdominals
- Lengthen spine
- Relax shoulders.

Coaching points

- Tighten the abdominal muscles
- Contract the abdominals to start the movement and lift the shoulders
- Keep the neck relaxed and looking forwards, following the movement of the rest of the spine
- Control the movement upwards and downwards.

For twisting sit-ups

- Rotate only as far as is comfortable, and without lifting the lower back off the floor
- Reverse the movement under control
- Ease the shoulder towards the knee rather than pulling the head over too far.

Progressions/Adaptations/Variations

- Repetitions; arm leverage; rate
- Perform with one leg on ball and other raised for variation.

Exercise 11.40	Reverse Curls – floor-lying with ball held between legs

Purpose

This exercise will work the muscles at the front of the trunk (rectus abdominis). Gripping the ball between the legs will work the inner thigh muscles (adductors).

Starting position and instructions

- Lying on floor, raise knees over hips and grip ball between legs
- Hollow the abdominals
- Lengthen spine
- Relax shoulders.

Coaching points:

- Contract the abdominals to raise the buttocks and create pelvic tilt action
- Take care not to swing the legs
- Take care not to hollow the lower back
- Do not allow the legs to travel out too far away from the central line of the body.

Progressions/Adaptations/Variations

Repetitions and rate.

Exercise 11.41	Rear leg raises – lying prone on the ball

Purpose

This exercise will work the buttock muscles (gluteus maximus).

Starting position and instructions

- Lie face down on the ball
- Hands on floor at shoulder-width-and-a-half apart with elbows extended
- Position hips on the ball with feet on floor (easier), *or* thighs on the ball, balancing (moderate), *or* feet on ball, balancing (harder)
- Maintain a neutral pelvic alignment and contract abdominals
- Raise one leg to just above hip-height, ensuring that a straight spine is maintained
- Lower down under control
- Perform the desired number of repetitions.

Coaching points

- Raise the leg under control
- Keep the abdominals pulled in tight and take care not to hollow the back
- Take care not to swing the leg.

Progressions/Adaptations/Variations

- Repetitions; rate; start position
- Option of double leg raise.

Exercise 11.42	Reciprocal reach – lying prone on the ball

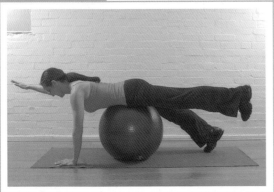

Purpose

This exercise will work the muscles of the buttocks (gluteus maximus) and the back of the shoulder/upper back (posterior deltoid and trapezius).

Starting position and instructions

- Lie face down on the ball
- Place hands shoulder-width-and-a-half apart on floor with elbows extended
- Position hips on the ball with feet on floor (easier), *or* thighs on the ball, balancing (moderate), *or* feet on ball, balancing (harder)
- Maintain a neutral pelvic alignment and contract abdominals
- Select one of the options listed in progressions/adaptations/variations, below.

Coaching points

- Raise arm and/or leg under control (see options)
- Keep the abdominals pulled in tight and take care not to hollow the back
- Lower down under control
- Perform the desired number of repetitions.

Progressions/Adaptations/Variations

- Lift one hand off the floor about one inch
- Lift one arm and extend in front of eye line
- Lift one leg (as per gluteal raise)
- Lift one arm and opposite leg.

Exercise 11.43	Back extensions – lying prone on the ball

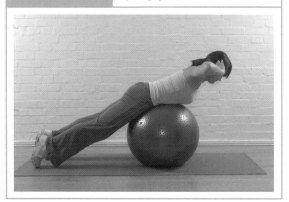

Purpose

This exercise will work the muscles that run along the length of the spine (erector spinae).

Starting position and instructions

- Lie on the ball face down and walk hands forwards to position body so that centre of the body rests across ball with feet touching the floor at hip-width. Hands should be able to reach and touch the floor slightly in front of the ball
- Maintain neutral pelvis with abdominals hollowed
- Lengthen the spine
- Shoulders should be relaxed, away from ears.

Coaching points

- Place hands either at side of head or on buttocks
- Lower the chest towards the floor and raise up to a slight hyperextension
- Keep the neck in line with rest of the spine
- Lift to a comfortable height
- Control the movement and breathe comfortably throughout.

Progressions/Adaptations/Variations

- Position of hands alters leverage
- Vary repetitions, rate and range of motion.

Exercise 11.44	Press-ups – lying prone on the ball

Purpose

This exercise will work the muscles at the front of the chest and shoulder (the pectorals and anterior deltoid) and the muscles at the back of the upper arm (triceps).

Starting position and instructions

- Hands on floor at shoulder-width-a-and half apart with elbows extended
- Position hips on the ball with feet on floor (easier), *or* thighs on the ball, balancing (moderate), *or* feet on ball, balancing (harder)
- Maintain a neutral pelvic alignment and contract abdominals
- Bend and straighten the elbows using press-up action.

Coaching points

- Keep the abdominals pulled in tight and the back straight
- Keep the whole of the spine and neck in line
- Ensure the elbows fully extend but do not lock
- Keep the body weight forwards and over the shoulders to maximise the resistance.

Progressions/Adaptations/Variations

- Body position on ball (hips, thighs, feet)
- Repetitions and rate.

Exercise 11.45	Prone flyes – lying prone on the ball

Purpose

This exercise will work the muscles in the middle of the back (trapezius).

Starting position and instructions

- Lie on the ball face down and walk hands forwards to position body so that centre of body rests across ball with feet touching the floor at hip-width. Hands should be able to reach and touch the floor slightly in front of the ball
- Maintain neutral pelvis with abdominals hollowed
- Lengthen the spine
- Shoulders should be relaxed, away from ears
- Keep arms positioned out to the side of the body.

Coaching points

- Raise and lower the arms under control
- Keep the abdominals pulled in tight
- Keep the elbows slightly bent
- Initiate the movement from the middle of the back by sliding the shoulder blades towards the buttocks
- Take care not to let the arms initiate and dictate the movement, but use the arms as resistance.

Progressions/Adaptations/ Variations

- To make the exercise easier, start with the hands at the side of the buttocks and gently lift the shoulders upwards, sliding the shoulder blades back and down
- Vary the speed, repetitions
- Use light dumbbells.

Exercise 11.46	Upright row – seated on ball

Purpose

This exercise will work the muscles at the front of the shoulder (anterior deltoid), the front of the upper arm (the biceps and brachialis) and the top of the back (the trapezius).

Starting position and instructions

- Sit centrally on the ball, feet on floor, with knees bent at hip-width
- Buttocks should be higher than knees
- Assume pelvis-neutral position (sitting on the sitting bones with pubic bone and hip bones in alignment)
- Keep abdominals hollowed and pulled in
- Lengthen spine so that ears, shoulders and hips are in line
- Keep shoulders relaxed and down
- Look forwards
- Dead-lift the dumbbells and sit upright.

Coaching points

- Position dumbbells at side of ball, palms face body
- Raise dumbbells level to chest, elbows lead, keep close to body
- Movement controlled.

Progressions/Adaptations/ Variations

- Vary the resistance, rate and repetitions
- Perform with alternate-leg seated calf raise
- Perform with alternating leg extension.

Exercise 11.47	Biceps curl – seated on ball

Purpose

This exercise will work the muscles at the front of the upper arm (the biceps and brachialis).

Starting position and instructions

- Sit centrally on the ball, feet on floor, with knees bent at hip-width
- Buttocks should be higher than knees
- Assume pelvis-neutral position (sitting on the sitting bones with pubic bone and hip bones in alignment)
- Keep abdominals hollowed and pulled in
- Lengthen spine so that ears, shoulders and hips are in line
- Keep shoulders relaxed and down
- Look forwards
- Dead-lift the dumbbells and sit upright.

Coaching points

- Raise and lower the dumbbells under control, in an arc-like motion
- Keep the wrist fixed and straight
- Keep the elbows and upper arm close to the body
- The lower arm should be the only body part moving
- Avoid locking the elbow.

Progressions/Adaptations/ Variations

- Vary the resistance, rate and repetitions
- Perform with alternate-leg seated calf raise
- Perform with alternating leg extension.

Exercise 11.48	Dumbbell lateral raise or front raise – seated on ball

Purpose

This exercise will work the shoulder muscles, the deltoids.

Starting position and instructions

- Sit centrally on the ball, feet on floor, with knees bent at hip-width
- Buttocks should be higher than knees
- Assume pelvis-neutral position (sitting on the sitting bones with pubic bone and hip bones in alignment)
- Keep abdominals hollowed and pulled in
- Lengthen spine so that ears, shoulders and hips are in line
- Keep shoulders relaxed and down
- Look forwards
- Dead-lift the dumbbells and sit upright.

Coaching points

- Raise and lower arms to side of the body; keep the wrist fixed
- Keep the elbow slightly bent
- Rotate the dumbbells as they are lifted so that the thumbs tilt forwards
- Keep the movement controlled.

Progressions/Adaptations/ Variations

- Vary the resistance, rate and repetitions
- Perform with alternate-leg seated calf raise
- Perform with alternating leg extension
- Raise to front to emphasise work for anterior deltoid.

Exercise 11.49	Calf raise and leg extension – seated on ball

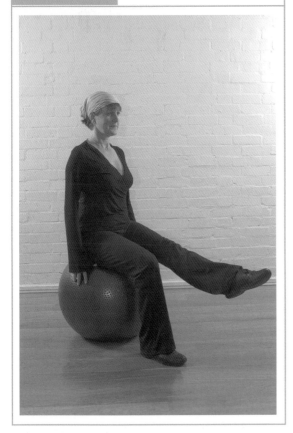

Purpose

Calf raise will work the soleus muscle. Leg extension will work the quadriceps muscle group.

Starting position and instructions

- Sit centrally on the ball, feet on floor, with knees bent at hip width.
- Buttocks should be higher than knees
- Assume pelvis-neutral position (sitting on the sitting bones with pubic bone and hip bones in alignment)

- Keep abdominals hollowed and pulled in
- Lengthen spine so that ears, shoulders and hips are in line
- Keep shoulders relaxed and down
- Look forwards
- Dead-lift the dumbbells and sit upright.

Coaching points

For calf raise

- Tighten abdominals to fix position and balance
- Raise on to ball of foot
- Lift and lower heel under control.

For leg extension

- Tighten abdominals to fix position
- Lift foot and extend knee to straight position without locking
- Lower under control
- Keep abdominals pulled in.

Progressions/Adaptations/Variations

- Can place hands at side of ball to assist balance initially
- Perform single or double leg calf raise
- Calf raise can be progressed to leg extension
- Can perform with upper body resistance exercises to add complexity
- Can perform in roll down bridge position – lying supine on ball.

Exercise 11.50	Overhead triceps press – seated on ball

Purpose

This exercise will work the muscles at the back of the upper arm (triceps).

Starting position and instructions

- Sit on the ball, feet hip-width apart
- Hold a dumbbell with both hands
- Raise the dumbbell overhead and fix in position
- Lower the dumbbell behind the head, bending at elbows
- Straighten the arms to return the dumbbell overhead.

Coaching Points

- Shoulders relaxed and away from ears
- Abdominals pulled in
- Upright posture
- Fully bend and straighten arms without locking elbows
- Keep elbows close to head.

Progressions/Adaptations/ Variations

- Use single arm to hold dumbbell
- Vary speed, repetitions and resistance to accommodate individuals.

Exercise 11.51	Shoulder press – seated on ball

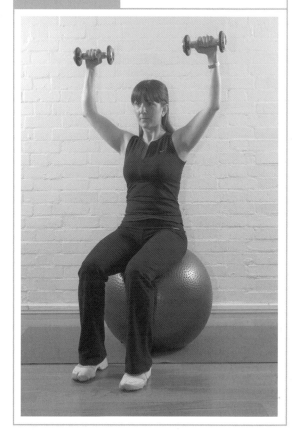

Purpose

This exercise will work the muscles at the back of the upper arm (triceps), shoulders (deltoids) and upper back (upper trapezius).

Starting position and instructions

- Sit on the ball, feet hip-width apart
- Hold a dumbbell in each hand
- Raise the dumbbells overhead into start position for shoulder press (elbows level with shoulders and wrist above elbows)
- Raise the dumbbells above head, straightening the elbows
- Lower under control.

Coaching Points

- Keep shoulders relaxed and away from ears
- Keep abdominals pulled in
- Fully bend and straighten arms without locking elbows.

Progressions/Adaptations/ Variations

- Use single arm shoulder press
- Use alternate arm shoulder press
- Vary speed, repetitions and resistance to accommodate individuals.

Exercise 11.52	Roll down – transition from seated to lying on ball

Purpose

This exercise can be used to get the body in position for exercises lying on the ball or as an exercise in its own right. As the latter, it assists improvement of mobility through the spine and strengthens the core abdominal muscles.

Starting position and instructions

- Sit centrally on the ball, feet on floor, with knees bent at hip-width
- Buttocks should be higher than knees
- Assume pelvis-neutral position (sitting on the sitting bones with pubic bone and hip bones in alignment)
- Tilt pelvis so that lower spine curls slightly
- Steadily walk feet away so that spine rolls down the ball
- End position should enable shoulder girdle to be resting on ball with feet on floor, knees over ankles and pelvis in neutral
- Roll up and reverse action using equal control.

Coaching points

- Roll down and roll up allowing each vertebra to make contact with ball
- For the end position, contract gluteals and abdominals to hold neutral position.

Progressions/Adaptations/ Variations

- Can place hands at side of ball to assist balance initially
- Can perform with calf raise or leg extension in end position.

Exercise 11.53	Chest press – lying supine on ball with feet on floor

Purpose

This exercise will work the muscles at the front of the chest (pectorals), the muscles at the front of the shoulder (the anterior deltoids) and the muscles at the back of the upper arm (the triceps).

Starting position and instructions

- Sit on ball, dead-lift dumbbells and hold level with chest (alternatively, use a spotter to pass dumbbells when in lying position)
- Roll down to get into lying position
- Position back centrally on the ball with the feet on floor and knees bent
- Maintain pelvis-neutral position
- Keep abdominals hollowed
- Lengthen spine and keep shoulders relaxed.

Coaching points:

- Knuckles should be facing upwards and the wrist be fixed
- Keep abdominals pulled in tight and take care not to hollow the back
- Move the dumbbells in a straight line, level with the chest
- Do not lock elbows
- Keep the movement smooth and under control.

Progressions/Adaptations/ Variations

Vary repetitions, resistance and rate of exercise. Performing this exercise with shoulder girdle placed on ball will demand greater stability and balance.

Exercise 11.54	Bent arm pullover – lying supine on ball with feet on floor

Purpose

This exercise will work the muscles at the front of the chest (pectorals) and the muscles at the side of the back (latissimus dorsi).

Starting position and instructions

- Sit on ball, dead-lift dumbbells and hold level with chest (alternatively, use a spotter to pass dumbbells when in position)
- Roll down to get into lying position and position back centrally on the ball with the feet on floor and knees bent
- Maintain pelvis-neutral position
- Lengthen spine and keep shoulders relaxed.

Coaching points

- Hold the dumbbells with elbows into sides of body at right angles
- Contract abdominals to maintain neutral pelvis
- Keeping the elbows bent, raise the arms in an arc-like motion to lift the dumbbells over the head and towards the floor
- Take care not to hollow the back, especially as the bar moves over the head and towards the floor
- Keep the elbows bent and pressed inwards (not splaying out)
- Breathe in a controlled manner throughout the exercise.

Progressions/Adaptations/ Variations

- Perform without weights to rehearse alignment
- Vary repetitions, rate and resistance
- Performing this exercise with shoulder girdle placed on ball will demand greater stability and balance.

Exercise 11.55	Lying triceps extension – lying supine on ball with feet on floor

Purpose

This exercise will work the muscles at the back of the upper arms (triceps).

Starting position and instructions

- Sit on ball and dead-lift dumbbells, and hold level with chest (alternatively, use a spotter to pass dumbbells when in position)
- Roll down to get into lying position
- Position back centrally on the ball with the feet on floor and knees bent
- Maintain pelvis-neutral position
- Keep abdominals hollowed
- Lengthen spine and keep shoulders relaxed.

Coaching points

- When in position, lift dumbbells overhead, arms extended
- Keep elbows in (not splaying); lower the dumbbell level with the bridge of the nose
- Return to upright position under control
- Keep the wrists and elbows fixed throughout the movement
- Keep the abdominals pulled in tight and take care not to hollow the back
- Straighten the arms fully but without locking the elbows.

Progressions/Adaptations/ Variations

- Perform without weights to rehearse the movement
- Vary repetitions, rate and resistance
- For advanced and more flexible participants,

take the bar down over the head. This will provide a greater range of motion and target the longer head of the triceps muscle
- Performing this exercise with shoulder girdle placed on ball will demand greater stability and balance.

Exercise 11.56	Lying dumbbell flyes – lying supine on ball with feet on floor

Purpose

This exercise will work the chest muscles (pectorals).

Starting position and instructions

- Sit on ball and dead-lift dumbbells, and hold level with chest (alternatively, use a spotter to pass dumbbells when in position)
- Roll down to get into lying position and position back centrally on the ball with the feet on floor and knees bent
- Maintain pelvis-neutral position
- Keep abdominals hollowed
- Lengthen spine and keep shoulders relaxed.

Coaching points

- When in position, press the dumbbells to the ceiling and level with the chest, palms face inwards
- Keep elbows unlocked and the arm fixed in this position
- Lower the dumbbells out to each side of the body, parallel to the floor
- Return the dumbbells back in towards the body
- Move the dumbbells under control
- Keep the abdominals pulled in tight and take care not to hollow the back

- Keep the wrist, elbow and shoulder in line throughout the movement
- Keep the wrist fixed and the elbows unlocked.

Progressions/Adaptations/ Variations

- Rehearse the movement without weights
- Vary repetitions, rate and resistance
- Performing this exercise with shoulder girdle placed on ball will demand greater stability and balance.

Exercise 11.57	Plank using core ball – lying prone, elbows on ball and feet on floor

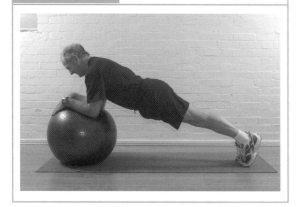

Purpose

This exercise will work the core muscles (transversus abdominis). Other muscles will work in a fixating capacity to hold the position.

Starting position and instructions

- From a kneeling position, rest the forearms on the ball, positioning shoulders over elbows

- Extend one leg back straight with ball of foot resting on floor
- Find pelvis-neutral position and contract abdominals
- Extend other leg back with ball of foot resting on floor
- Ensure body is extended.

Coaching points

- Keep the abdominals pulled in tight and spine aligned
- Relax shoulders away from ears and allow shoulder blades to slide down towards buttocks
- Keep the elbow and shoulder aligned
- Keep the knees unlocked
- Keep the head in line with the rest of the body.

Progressions/Adaptations/ Variations

- Hold for a longer duration
- Raise alternate legs and hold off the floor
- Place hands on the ball and perform with straight arms
- Progress straight arm plank to a narrow hand press-up with hands on ball.

PART FOUR

WORKING WITH DIFFERENT GROUPS AND OUTDOOR CIRCUITS

BISHOP BURTON COLLEGE

INTRODUCTION

This section identifies factors that need to be considered prior to taking a circuit session for the general population, and also for specialist groups such as older adults and sportspeople.

A needs analysis for exercises is provided for all groups with example lesson plans for a complete circuit training session to meet different needs and abilities for both indoor and outdoor circuits.

To assist with planning a progressive circuit training programme for any group, the following 'SMART' goal-setting strategy can be used:

S	**Specific** Make the aim and goals of the circuit specific and appropriate for the needs identified	**Example goals and aims of the circuit:** To challenge muscular endurance of the abdominals and back To develop cardiovascular fitness To develop muscular strength and endurance of all muscles.
M	**Measurable** Ensure the goals of the circuit can be measured to enable individuals to monitor their achievement and progress	**Measurable criteria:** Choice of exercise (complexity, intensity and type) Starting repetitions Starting resistance Number of exercises Number of circuits Work and rest ratio Use of equipment Duration of the whole circuit Frequency of circuit training sessions (per week).

A	**Achievable** Ensure that the measurable activities are achievable by all participants	**Achievable criteria:** Related to individual needs and differences (age, gender, sports-specific etc.) Have alternative options for all exercises to accommodate different levels and needs when working with groups of mixed ability Have progressive options for all exercises to accommodate different levels and needs when working with groups of mixed ability
R	**Realistic** The session must contain a range of alternatives and progressions for different abilities	**Realistic criteria:** Progression needs to account for individual differences Anticipated achievement and outcomes for individuals must be realistic and match their ability for the specified time period Circuit cards need to show different exercise options and/or repetition options Teaching style needs to reflect requirements of different individuals when working with groups of mixed ability, e.g. use of demonstrations, coaching points, motivation strategies etc.
T	**Timed** Progression of the circuit should be planned over an established period of time	**Timed criteria:** Within a timed progressive plan (e.g. 15-week time period) adjustments need to be made to account for individual differences and needs when working with groups of mixed abilities Each individual will progress at their own rate. For example, at the end of a 15-week programme, a realistic and achievable outcome for one person might be to perform X number of full press-ups. For another individual, a realistic and achievable outcome would be to perform X number of three-quarter press-ups.

GENERAL POPULATIONS

12

To design a safe and effective circuit training session, it is necessary to conduct a needs analysis for the specific exercising group. The following considerations need to be addressed:

- thorough pre-screening to identify any specific injuries that need to be either referred to the GP or accommodated for within the session
- the current fitness level of the exercising group and individuals within the group. How flexible are they? How much muscular strength and endurance do they have? How long can they sustain aerobic/anaerobic activities? What level of intensity (target heart rate/RPE) and what type of activities push the individual closer towards their anaerobic threshold?
- the primary aims and goals of the session for that specific group (i.e. improve cardiovascular fitness, improve health and wellbeing, etc.)

- the aims and goals of individuals within the group, and whether they can be accommodated. For example, losing weight, meeting new people and trying a new activity may all be different goals
- the current lifestyles of individuals, e.g. how active are they at work or at home? Are they eating an appropriate diet, etc.?

Spending time on this analysis will ensure that the initial circuit session designed will be safe, effective and enjoyable. However, it is clear from the information outlined above that no two individuals within any specific group will be identical. Therefore, the teacher will need to be ready to think on their feet and adapt the session and specific exercises to meet certain individual needs. A sample needs analysis is provided in Table 12.1. For further guidelines on progressing a circuit and each component of fitness, please refer to Parts One and Two of this book.

Table 12.1	Needs analysis and guidelines for the general population		
	Beginner	**Intermediate**	**Advanced**
General aims and goals	Developing skills and correct exercise technique Building an all-round base level of fitness in all components	Building repertoire of exercises Continued focus on maintaining safe and effective exercise technique	Maintenance fitness training programme Continued maintenance of correct exercise technique

Table 12.1	Needs analysis and guidelines for the general population cont.		
	Improving health status	Building further on base level of fitness	Developing exercise repertoire further Identifying other modes of exercise/introducing cross-training
Frequency of exercise and training sessions, and other daily activities	Building up to three training sessions per week Increase activities for daily life, i.e. vigorous housework, walk to the shops, etc.	Minimum of three training sessions per week Other exercise alternatives can be explored Continue developing activities for daily living	Three to five sessions Cross-train to vary exercise programme Maintain daily living activities
Intensity	Low	Moderate	Moderate to high
Resistance	Lower	Moderate	Comparatively higher
Rate control	Slower	Moderate	Optimal speed, maintaining control
Range of motion (ROM) (NB: always work to individual's existing range of motion)	Generally smaller ROM	Increased ROM	Full potential ROM
Time	45 mins	45 mins to one hour	One hour
Type	Circuit	Circuit	Circuit
Other types of activity that can be recommended	Walking Swimming Cycling Other beginners' exercise programmes Other beginners' stretching programmes	Jogging Cycling More energetic swimming Weight training Other intermediate exercise programmes	Jogging Weight training Training for a specific event (e.g. 10k run)

LESSON PLANS FOR GENERAL FITNESS

13

The groups dealt with in this section have different fitness levels. These are categorised as beginner, intermediate and advanced. However, teachers should recognise that such terminology is generalised. For instance, a participant may have a good level of muscular strength but limited flexibility and/or cardiovascular fitness. Thus, they could be categorised as advanced for the former fitness component and a beginner for the latter two components. The lesson plans provided are intended as a guide. They can be adapted in many ways to suit the needs of the group and the nature of the circuit.

Table 13.1	General fitness warm-up for beginners	
Timing	**Exercise/activity**	**Purpose**
30 secs	Walk anywhere in area (6.11)	General pulse-raising
1 min	Continue walking, adding shoulder lifts and shoulder rolls (6.1)	Shoulder mobility and general pulse-raising
30 secs	In place leg curls (6.5)	Knee mobility and pulse-raising
30 secs	In place knee lifts (6.6)	Hip mobility and pulse-raising
2 mins 30 secs	Repeat all of above with larger stride and larger range of motion	As above
30 secs	In place side twists (6.3)	Mobilising spine
30 secs	In place side bends (6.2)	Mobilising spine
1 min	Brisk walk in circle, changing direction and building intensity to a light skip	General pulse-raising
30 secs	Squat in place and biceps curls (11.26)	Mobilising knees and elbows, and general pulse-raising; practising arm line for biceps curls

Table 13.1	General fitness warm-up for beginners cont.	
30 secs	Walk briskly anywhere, pushing arms forwards – press-up action	General pulse-raising and practising arm movement for press-up
Total time – 8 mins		
2 mins	Walk in a circle and strecth latissimus dorsi/pectorals and triceps (7.5/7.18/7.6)	Lengthening muscles
2 mins	March in place and rear lunges (9.19) into calf stretch right and left	
I min	Heel digs into back of thigh stretch right and left (7.1)	
I min	Squat in place into inner thigh stretch (7.4)	
30 secs	Quad stretch right and left using wall for balance	
Total time for stretch – 6.5 mins *Total time for warm-up – 14.5 mins*		
3–5 mins re-warmer	Re-warm and specific preparation for circuit. Use exercises on pp.68–71 and build intensity gradually	Introduce circuit stations, build heart rate slightly to level of circuit

Beginners

General fitness circuit training for beginners

Circuit One

- Six stations
- Muscular strength and endurance bias
- 30 secs on each exercise
- 10 secs rest between exercises
- Twice round circuit progressing to three times round or increase number of work stations
- Line approach and colour code to indicate different intensity levels
- Equipment – mats/barbells/dumbbells
- Total time = 8 mins progressing to 12 mins.

Circuit Two

- Eight stations
- Cardiovascular bias
- 30 secs on each exercise
- No rest. 30 secs active walk to next station and march in place before commencing next station
- 3 × around circuit progressing to 4 × around
- Corner approach
- Total time = 12 mins progressing to 16 mins.

Fig 13.1 Circuit One

Station 1 – Back raises	Station 4 – Curl-ups
Station 2 – Press-ups	Station 5 – Prone flyes
Station 3 – Dead-lift	Station 6– Biceps curls

Fig 13.2(a) Circuit Two – corner layout

Corner 1	Corner 3
Corner 2	Corner 4

Table 13.2 Circuit Two – exercise stations

	Circuit A	Circuit B
Corner 1	Half jacks	Squats
Corner 2	Front leg kicks	Knee lifts
Corner 3	Shuttle walks to diagonal corner	Gallops or side steps to diagonal corner and back
Corner 4	Backward lunges	Leg curls

NB: can progress to square layout with 8–10 stations per circuit, as in Fig. 13.2(b). Circuit stations can have cardiovascular bias, work for specific muscle groups, or be alternated within circuit, e.g. CV station/MSE station/CV station/MSE station, and so on.

Fig 13.2(b) Circuit Two – station layout

Station 1 Half jacks	Station 2 Sit-ups	Station 3 Knee lift	Station 4 Prone flyes
Shuttle walk/run Station 5	Back extension Station 6	Press-ups Station 7	Squats Station 8

Table 13.3	General fitness warm-down for beginners	
Timing	**Exercise/activity**	**Purpose**
1 min	Brisk walk/skip and chest press, rolling shoulders back	Maintain intensity of circuit. NB: depending on the nature of the preceding circuit, the intensity may need to commence at a slightly higher level
30 secs	Travelling side squats, four right and four left, and repeat (6.9)	Maintaining intensity
1 min 30 secs	Repeat above, reducing stride length and range of motion	Lowering intensity
1 min	Backward lunges (9.19) into calf stretch right and left	Lengthening muscles
1 min 30 secs	Walk anywhere and stretch latissimus dorsi/pectorals and triceps (7.5/7.18/7.6)	Lowering intensity and lengthening muscles
30 secs	Gentle walk around	Lowering intensity
1 min	Quad stretch (7.2) right and left, using wall for balance	Lengthening muscles
1 min 30 secs	Lying on floor, back of thigh stretch (7.10 or 7.14 seated)	
1 min	Seated inner thigh stretch (7.13)	
2 mins	Come to standing and walk gently anywhere, rolling shoulders (6.1)	Revitalise

Total time – 11.5 mins
NB: additional time needed to teach stretch positions and allow full recovery.

Intermediate

General fitness circuit training for intermediate-level participants

Circuit One

- Twelve stations – can add stations to build time of circuit
- Mixed muscular strength and endurance/ aerobic (alternate aerobic and MSE stations)
- 50 secs on each exercise
- 10 secs rest (change around to next station)
- Once around circuit
- Square format
- Total time = 12 mins – can go twice around as fitness increases.

Circuit Two

- Twelve stations
- Mixed muscular strength and endurance/aerobic (alternate aerobic and MSE stations)
- 30 secs on each exercise
- 30 active performance of shuttle walks/runs
- to opposite end of hall before moving on to next station
- Once around circuit, progressing to twice around or increase number of work stations
- Lined approach
- Total time = 12–24 mins.

Fig 13.3 Circuit One – Twelve-station square circuit

Station 1	Station 2	Station 3	Station 4
Press-ups	Squats	Curl-ups	Jumping jacks
Station 12			Station 5
Shuttle runs			Back raises
Station 11			Station 6
Upright row			Spotty dogs
Station 10	Station 9	Station 8	Station 7
Knee lifts	Reverse curls	Step-ups	Biceps curls

Fig 13.4 Circuit Two – Twelve-station lined circuit

	Station 1 – Upright row with bands
	Station 2 – Curl-up and twist
Station 3 – Star jumps	
Station 4 – Triceps dips	
Station 5 – Lunges	
	Station 6 – Reverse curls
Station 7 – Press-ups	
Station 8 – Bent over row	
Station 9 – Squats	
	Station 10 – Biceps curls
Station 11 – Combined back raise and prone flye	
Station 12 – Press-ups	
	Perform shuttles*

*Shuttle runs/walks for 30 secs in-between stations

Table 13.4	General fitness warm-up for intermediate-level participants	
Timing	**Exercise/activity**	**Purpose**
1 min 30 secs	Walking in circle with shoulder lifts, shoulder rolls (6.1), and pressing arms forwards	Shoulder mobility, general pulse-raising and rehearsing arm lines for press-ups and biceps curls
1 min	Face into circle, perform leg curls (6.5), travelling forwards into centre of the circle with biceps curls (11.26) and knee lifts (6.6), travelling backwards to outside of circle	Mobilising knees, hips and elbows, general pulse-raising and rehearsing biceps curl arm action
2 mins 30 secs	Repeat all of the above with larger stride and larger range of motion	As above
30 secs	In place squat and side twists right (6.3), repeat and twist left	Mobilising spine and knee, and maintaining pulse-raising
1 min	In place side bends (6.2) and reach arms overhead – shoulder press (9.24)	Mobilising spine and rehearsing should press action
	Total time – 6 mins 30 secs	
1 min	Walking in a circle and stretching latissimus dorsi/pectorals and triceps (7.5/7.18/7.6)	Lengthening muscles
1 min	March in place and backward lunges (9.19) into calf stretch right and left (7.3)	
1 min	Heel digs into back of thigh stretch right and left (7.1)	
30 secs	Squat in place into inner thigh stretch (7.4)	
30 secs	Quad stretch right and left	
	Total time for stretch – 4 mins *Total time for warm-up – 10 mins 30 secs*	
3–5 mins re-warmer	Re-warm and specific preparation for circuit. Use exercises on pp. 68–71	Introduce circuit stations and build heart rate to level of circuit

NB: could adapt by using a colour-coded repetition circuit, e.g. participants choose repetition range (8–20) appropriate to their ability for each station. Once station is complete, participants perform shuttle walks or runs until whole group have finished circuit. Whole group then move on to the next station.

Table 13.5	General fitness warm-down for intermediate-level participants	
Timing	**Exercise/activity**	**Purpose**
1 min 30 secs	Moderate pace jog in a circle, reducing to a skip	Maintain intensity of circuit, gradually reducing pace to lower intensity. NB: depending on the nature of the preceding circuit, the intensity may need to commence at a slightly higher level
1 min 30 secs	Gentle gallops to right and left, facing into and out of circuit, reducing to side squats	Progressively lowering intensity
1 min	Backward lunges into calf stretch (7.3) and hip flexor stretch, right to left	Lowering intensity and lengthening muscles
1 min	Walk anywhere and stretch latissimus dorsi/pectorals and triceps (7.5/7.18/7.6)	Lowering intensity and lengthening muscles
30 secs	Quad stretch (7.2) right and left, using wall for balance	Lengthening muscles
1 min	Lying on floor, back of thigh stretch (7.10 or 7.14 seated)	
1 min	Seated inner thigh stretch (7.13) and seated abductor stretch (7.13)	
1 min 30 secs	Come to standing and walk gently anywhere, rolling shoulders (6.1) Hump and hollow (6.4) into back stretch (7.17), and walk around 'High-five' as you meet other participants, and say 'Well done!'	Revitalise
Total time – 9 mins		
NB: additional stretches included to compensate for anticipated harder workout		

Advanced

General fitness circuit training for advanced participants

Circuit One – part one

- Twelve stations
- Muscular strength and endurance bias

- 30 secs on each exercise
- No rest (change around)
- Working clockwise
- Twice around circuit
- Switch to aerobic circuit when complete.

Table 13.6	General fitness warm-up for advanced-level participants	
Timing	**Exercise/activity**	**Purpose**
1 min 30 secs	Brisk walk around area. Continue moving around, adding leg curls (6.5). Continue moving around and changing direction, adding knee lifts (6.6)	General pulse-raising and mobility for knees and hips
30 secs	Stationary side bends (6.2) and side twists (6.3)	Spine mobility
45 secs	Brisk walk in any direction, rolling shoulders	General pulse-raising and shoulder mobility
45 secs	Stationary steps back, pushing arms forwards	General pulse-raising
1 min	Brisk walk anywhere, increasing arm swing	
30 secs	Stationary squats (9.11) – half range of motion	General pulse-raising and knee mobility
Total time – 5 mins for mobility pulse-raising **Repeat sections if cold environment**		
30 secs	Walking with back of the upper arm stretch (7.6)	Pulse-raising and lengthening muscles
45 secs	Backward lunges (9.19) into calf lunges combined with chest stretch (7.7) and upper back stretch	
30 secs	Brisk walk with knee lifts (6.6) and pulling arms down	

Table 13.6	General fitness warm-up for advanced-level participants cont.	
30 secs	Stationary quad stretch	Lengthening muscles
30 secs	Brisk walk anywhere, adding leg curls (6.5)	Pulse-raising and lengthening muscles
30 secs	Stationary back of the thigh stretch (7.10)	Lengthening muscles
30 secs	Walking forward lunges into hip flexor stretch (7.15)	Pulse-raising and lengthening muscles
45 secs	Squats into stationary inner thigh stretch (7.13), and hump and hollow (6.4) into erector spinae stretch	Lengthening muscles
Total time – 4.5 mins for preparatory stretches **Total warm-up time – 9.5 mins**		
Specific re-warm for aerobic (cardiovascular) and MSE circuit	Walk anywhere with chest press arms Step backs with shoulder press (9.24) Brisk walk and lateral raise arms Stationary squat (9.11) and front raise arms Low-level jog in any direction with arm swings Fuller range of motion squat and biceps curls (11.26) Stationary lunge with triceps extension Jogging any direction Spotty dogs (9.3) Jogging squats and calf raise (11.24)	Re-warm and rehearse circuit stations. Introduce stations
Total time – 4–5 mins for re-warm		

Fig 13.5 (a) Circuit One – Twelve-station square circuit

Station 1 Back extensions	Station 2 Lunges	Station 3 Biceps curls	Station 4 Abdominal curls and twists
Station 12 Triceps dips			Station 5 Dead-lift
Station 11 The plank			Station 6 Calf raises
Station 10 Upright rows	Station 9 Alternate leg squat thrusts	Station 8 Reverse curls	Station 7 Press-ups

Circuit One – part two

- Six stations
- Aerobic/cardiovascular bias
- 60 secs on each exercise
- No rest (change around)
- Line approach
- Anticlockwise, once around
- Switch to muscular strength and endurance circuit when complete.

Circuit Two

- Three stations
- Muscular strength and endurance bias
- 30 secs on each exercise/2 mins per body area
- Move continuously from one exercise to another
- Overload/supersets approach
- Total time = 6 mins.

Fig 13.5(b) Circuit One – Six-station lined circuit

Station 1 – Jumping jacks

Station 2 – Travelling lunges

Station 3 – Leg curls

Station 4 – Power squats

Station 5 – Shuttle runs

Station 6 – Step-ups

NB: half the group can perform MSE circuit while the other half perform CV circuit

Fig 13.6 Circuit Two

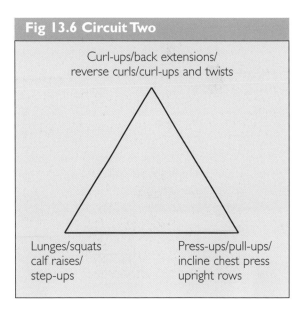

Curl-ups/back extensions/ reverse curls/curl-ups and twists

Lunges/squats calf raises/ step-ups

Press-ups/pull-ups/ incline chest press upright rows

Table 13.7	General fitness warm-down for advanced-level participants	
Timing	**Exercise/activity**	**Purpose**
1 min	Jogging anywhere, punching arms forwards and upwards, then pressing arms forwards	Maintain intensity of circuit
30 secs	Stationary squats (9.11) and biceps curls (11.26)	Lowering intensity
30 secs	Reduced pace jog	
30 secs	Lunges – half range of motion (9.19)	
1 min	Brisk walking	
30 secs	Small range of motion squat	
Total time for pulse-lowering – 4 mins		
1 min	Backward lunges (9.19) into calf stretch (7.3) combined with chest stretch (7.7). Follow with hip flexor stretch (7.15) right and left	Lengthening muscles
1 min	Walk anywhere and stretch latissimus dorsi and triceps (7.5/7.6)	Lowering intensity and lengthening muscles
30 secs	Quad stretch (7.2) right and left, using wall for balance	Lengthening muscles
1 min	Lying on floor – back of thigh stretch (7.10 or 7.14, seated)	
30 secs	Lying gluteal stretch	
1 min	Seated inner thigh stretch (7.13) and seated abductor stretch (7.13)	
Total time for post-workout stretches – 5 mins		
1 min 30 secs	Come to standing and gently walk anywhere, rolling shoulders (6.1). Hump and hollow into back stretch (7.17) and walk around. 'High-five' as you meet other participants, and say 'Well done!'	Revitalise
Total time for complete warm-down/cool-down component – 10.5 mins		
Additional stretches included to compensate for anticipated harder workout		

Between circuits – CV work

Continuous performance of a combination of different exercises performed on command while running around hall:

- star jumps
- spotty dogs
- front kicks
- rear lunges
- knee lifts
- leg curls
- side lunges
- no rest
- command circuit approach

Total time – 4 mins
Total number of circuits – 2–3
Total work time on circuit – 20–30 mins.

General population – Abdominal and back circuit

Table 13.8	Guidelines for warming up and cooling down for abdominal and back circuit
Warm-up guidelines for an abdominal and back circuit	**Cool-down guidelines for an abdominal and back circuit**
Pulse raising Light, low-intensity activities, e.g. Marching on the spot Walking Squats Knee bends	**Pulse lowering** Light, low-intensity activities, e.g. Marching on the spot Walking Squats Knee bends
Mobility Focus on spine and trunk, e.g. Side bends Trunk twists Hump and hollow spine in standing position Pelvic tilts	**Mobility** Include additional mobility exercises for spine and trunk, e.g. Seated side bends Seated trunk rotations Pelvic tilts Cat stretch – rounding and flattening back Floor lying – roll up to bridge
Stretching: Focus on trunk and mid section, e.g. Side of body stretch	**Stretching:** Focus on trunk and mid section, e.g. Lying oblique stretch Seated side of body stretch Cat stretch – on hands and knees and humping spine Erector spinae stretch – lying on floor holding knees towards chest

Table 13.9	Example exercises and circuit plan for different fitness levels			
	Beginner	**Intermediate**	**Advanced**	**Suggestions for Progression**
No of circuits:	1–2	2	2–3	Increase number of circuits
Work:Rest Guidelines	30:30	40:20	50:10	Increase work time and decrease rest time
Number of exercises	4–8	8–12	12–16	Increase number of stations and use harder exercises
Station 1	Curl-up	Curl-up	Curl-up	Hands on thighs Hands across chest Hands side of head
Station 2	Back extension	Back extension	Back extension	Hands on floor Hands side of body Hands side of head
Station 3	Reverse curl	Reverse curl	Reverse curl	Heels on buttocks Knees fixed at 90 degrees Legs extended over belly button
Station 4	Trunk twists	Trunk twists	Trunk twists	Hands on thighs Hands across chest Hands side of head
Station 5	Core ball balance Seated on ball – pelvic tilt Can progress to repeat stations 1–5 with beginners working on technique. As progression occurs introduce additional exercises	Core ball balance Seated on ball – heel raise	Core ball balance Seated on ball – leg extension	Pelvic tilt Calf raise Leg extension
Station 6		Crunch: Reverse curl with curl up	Crunch: Reverse curl with curl up	Alternate one then other Perform both together

Table 13.9	Example exercises and circuit plan for different fitness levels cont.			
Station 7		Trunk twist and cycle legs at 45 degrees	Trunk twist and cycle legs at 45 degrees	Hold knees bent at 90 degrees and crunch (no cycle) Cycle legs without moving upper body and fixate abdominals Twist and cycle
Station 8		Roll down on ball	Roll down on ball	Hold position Heel raise while holding position Knee extension while holding position
Station 9		Curl-up on ball	Curl-up on ball	Hands on thighs Hands across chest Hands side of head
Station 10		Curl-up and twist on ball	Curl-up and twist on ball	Hands on thighs Hands across chest Hands side of head
Station 11		Bridge on ball	Bridge on ball	Bridge and roll
Station 12		Reciprocal reach on ball	Reciprocal reach on ball	Hands lift Arm extends Leg extends Arm and opposite leg extend

CIRCUIT TRAINING FOR OLDER ADULTS

14

This chapter discusses the effects of ageing on the body, the benefits of circuit training for an older adult, and an appropriate session structure. It also outlines how to adapt each component of the session to accommodate some of the requirements of an older exerciser. Example session plans for the older adult, with suggestions from Keith Smith, are provided at the end of the chapter.

Benefits from physical activity can be obtained, no matter what age we start exercising. However, the rate at which we progress will be slightly slower when we are older and it will therefore take slightly longer for us to achieve and to notice improvements.

Older adults who have maintained an active lifestyle might be able to cope quite comfortably with a more demanding programme. Alternatively, frail, elderly groups may find even a seated programme too much. Therefore, it is recommended that teachers remain aware of the group and the individuals they are teaching. Furthermore, it should be recognised that the information that follows in this chapter in no way provides all the necessary information for teaching a seniors group. It should not be used to substitute attendance on a teacher training programme that deals with the needs of this specialist group in greater depth.

How does the ageing process affect our body?

Ageing has a significant affect on the body. The skeletal, muscular, cardiovascular, respiratory and nervous systems are all affected by the ageing process. Some of the changes that occur are outlined in Tables 14.1–14.4. Age-related changes generally begin to occur at 50 years of age, and make their mark at around 65 years of age. Whereas an inactive lifestyle and disuse of the muscles may contribute to the early onset of ageing, physical activity and regular use of the muscles can slow down the ageing process. It is therefore possible for an active 70- or 80-year-old to be in better shape and condition than an inactive 40-year-old. Awareness of the age-related changes will assist the circuit training teacher in adapting exercises accordingly.

How will movements need to be adapted?

The following is a brief list of how movements can be adapted to accommodate the problems identified in Table 14.1:

- Movements of the joints will need to be slower and more controlled
- Excessively high impact activities should not be undertaken
- Emphasis should be placed on working the muscles that will improve posture
- Increase joint mobilising activities

- Include strengthening exercises to improve bone density
- Specific adaptations may need to be made for those with specialist conditions (arthritis, etc.). Please consult a medical practitioner or physiotherapist if you are in doubt or require further information.

The following is a brief list of how movements can be adapted to accommodate the problems identified in Table 14.2:

- All movements will need to be slower
- More time will need to be allowed for directional changes
- Movement patterns will need to be simplified and repeated sequentially
- All activities will need to be less intense

- Greater emphasis should be placed on alignment and the maintenance of correct technique
- Explosive movements or high impact moves should not be included
- A lower number of repetitions of the same exercise will need to be performed, to prevent fatigue
- Specific activities to strengthen the pelvic floor muscles should also be included.

The following is a brief list of how movements can be adapted to accommodate the problems identified in Table 14.3:

- Activities will need to be less intense
- Activities may need to be performed for a shorter duration

Table 14.1	The effects of ageing on the skeletal system	
Effects of ageing	**Associated problems**
Decreased bone density (less calcium in the bones)	Brittle bones – osteoporosis Postural problems, such as spinal curvatures
Calcification (laying down of bone) of the cartilage in joints	Increased likelihood of joint-associated disease, such as arthritis
Decreased availability of synovial fluid (which lubricates the joints) in the joints	Less effective shock absorption by joints Stiff and less mobile joints

Table 14.2	The effects of ageing on the muscular system	
Effects of ageing	**Associated problems**
• Decreased efficiency of motor neurons (nerves transmitting messages to the muscles) • Decreased fast twitch muscle fibres (used during strength training and power activities) • Decreased concentration of myosin and actin (smallest muscle fibres) • Reduced capillarisation (poorer blood supply to muscles) • Increased connective tissue in the muscles • Reduced elasticity in ligaments and tendons	• Reduced movement speed • Less potential muscle strength, especially for fast-reaction movements • Loss of muscle tissue • Less potential muscle endurance • Less flexibility • Stiffer and less mobile joints • Weakened pelvic floor muscles

- Lower repetitions of intense movements to prevent fatigue
- Explosive or high intensity movements will be inappropriate
- Longer time will need to be spent preparing the body for activity, and for recovery after activity
- Further adaptations will need to be made for persons with specialist conditions (e.g. high blood pressure, etc.).

The following is a brief list of how movements can be adapted to accommodate the problems identified in Table 14.4:
- Movements will need to be simpler
- Movement patterns will need to be more repetitive, but without becoming too enduring

- Stable exercise positions will need to be provided
- Movements will need to be slower
- Further adaptations will need to be made for those with specialist conditions.

How should an older adults' programme be structured?

As with all other sessions, sufficient time should be spent warming up before the main activity and cooling down afterwards. A circuit training programme which trains all of the components of fitness is ideal. However, the duration and intensity of the whole session and each component part will need to be adapted for an

Table 14.3	The effects of ageing on the cardiovascular system
Effects of ageing	**Associated problems**
• Decreased gaseous exchange, elasticity of the lungs and flexibility of the thorax • Lower cardiac output and less efficient circulatory system • Reduced capillary network and oxygen delivered to cells • Increased blood pressure	• Reduced breathing rate and oxygen uptake • Lower maximal heart rate and slower recovery rate • Decreased tolerance to fatigue and waste products such as lactic acid • Increased likelihood of disease of the cardiovascular and respiratory system, e.g. atherosclorosis

Table 14.4	The effects of ageing on the nervous system
Effects of ageing	**Associated problems**
• Poor short-term memory • Balance impaired • Reduced number of messages from brain to body, due to death of nerve cells • Reduced number of neurons and increased grey matter	• Forget movement patterns more rapidly • Difficulty stabilising a position and maintaining balance • Reduced body awareness • Reduced movement speed • Increased likelihood of disease of the nervous system (e.g. Parkinson's disease)

older adults' programme. The complete session will need to be slightly shorter and of a lower and more moderate intensity. This is variable depending on the fitness of the group. Guidelines for the timing and duration of specialist programmes are outlined in Tables 14.5 and 14.11 (Chapter 14). More specific guidelines for selecting the appropriate activities for an older adults' programme are outlined in Table 14.5. A sample lesson plan for an appropriate circuit training programme is provided in Chapter 13.

Summary of personal information that needs to be gathered prior to teaching older adults

Pre-exercise assessment and more detailed information-gathering techniques should be used to ensure the circuit is planned at an appropriate intensity and meets the needs of the group. Information should be gathered regarding their:
- general activity levels (lifestyle)
- fitness levels
- skill levels
- specific medical conditions (GP referral should be requested if necessary)
- specific wants and needs.

Summary of environmental and equipment considerations that need to be accommodated when designing the circuit for the older adult

- Clear working floor area
- Circuit cards and equipment off the floor and visible
- Functional exercise stations related to daily life activity needs
- Postural stations

- Lower work-to-rest ratios at each station
- Isotonic muscle work (specific isometric muscle work)
- Effective alternatives
- Whole body approach
- Resources available
- Clearly printed circuit cards
- Avoid too many flexion exercises
- Balance exercise stations
- Consider functional loading when putting two exercises for same muscle group together, e.g. walking followed by step-ups.

General circuit training for active older adults

Circuit One

- Six to 10 stations achieving balanced whole body approach
- Encourage movements and exercises that resemble daily lifestyle activities. Maintain activity levels and functional movement. Improvements to fitness will be comparatively less for older populations
- Work ratio 20–40 secs depending on activity levels and fitness
- Rest ratio 10–20 secs. Participants could be encouraged to march in place between exercise stations
- One to two circuits
- Music can be used to make for a more social environment
- Total time = 5–15 mins.

Table 14.5	Adaptations to session components for an older adults' programme
Warm-up component	• more mobility exercises for each joint • more isolated mobility work for each joint • slower, more controlled mobility exercises to promote an easy but fuller range of motion • more mobility exercises for minor joints • more emphasis on exercise technique • less intense pulse-raising • less directional changes • slower movements • shorter levers • slower transitions • fewer stretches • easier and more stable, balanced positions • possibly fewer stretches, since some positions may be inappropriate • more care getting into and out of stretch positions
Cardiovascular training	• spend slightly longer on the re-warmer and cool-down phases, to allow training for a more gradual building up and slowing down of intensity • lower intensity cardiovascular exercises • duration of time at each station should be adapted to suit the ability of the group • slower movements • use an interval training approach combining low-intensity work with occasional short bursts of moderate-intensity activities. The frequency of more moderately paced activities will be dependent on the fitness of the group
Muscular strength and endurance exercises	• fewer repetitions of each exercise, therefore shorter time at each station • lower resistance • slower movements through the full range of motion • target postural muscles (quadriceps, hamstrings, erector spinae, abdominals, trapezius, calf muscles) • target muscles to assist with daily activities, e.g. triceps – for pushing oneself out of the bath; and biceps – for lifting and carrying objects • select more stable and comfortable positions • include stretches for each muscle once a specific exercise is completed (this will shorten time needed for cooling down)
Cool-down component	• shorter component • combine stretches with flowing movements to keep warm (i.e. smaller range of motion of stretches) • hold static stretches for less time • select positions which offer more support and assist balance

Table 14.6	General warm-up for active older adults	
Timing	**Exercise/activity**	**Purpose**
1 min	Walk anywhere in area (6.11)	General pulse-raising
1 min	March in place with shoulder rolls	Shoulder mobility and general pulse-raising
30 secs	Knee bends/shallow squats	Knee and hip mobility and general pulse-raising
30 secs	Walk in a circle	General pulse-raising
30 secs	In place leg curls (6.5)	Knee mobility and pulse-raising
30 secs	In place knee lifts (6.6)	Hip mobility and pulse-raising
4 mins	Repeat all of the above with larger stride and larger range of motion	As above
30 secs	In place side twists (6.3)	Spine mobility
30 secs	In place side bends (6.2)	
30 secs	Walk briskly anywhere	General pulse-raising
	Total time – 9 mins 30 secs	
2 mins	Walk in a circle and stretch latissimus dorsi/pectorals and triceps (7.5/7.18/7.6)	Lengthening muscles
2 mins	March in place and backward lunges (9.19) into calf stretch right and left (7.3)	
1 min	Heel digs into back of thigh stretch right and left (7.1)	
1 min	Squat in place into inner thigh stretch (7.4)	
30 secs	Quad stretch right and left, using wall for balance	
	Total time for stretching – 6 mins 30mins	
	Total time for warm-up – 16 mins	
	Next stage of session: re-warm and specific preparation for circuit	

Table 14.7	Circuit One
Exercise stations	**Alternatives**
1. Walking through crowds (use chairs scattered around room to assimilate people	1. Shuttle walks
2. Dead-lift (use lightly weighted shopping bags)	2. Half squat
3. Crossing the road	3. Step-up with wall support
4. Shoulder press	4. Lateral raise
5. Standing upright row	5. Single-arm row
6. Standing calf raise and toe-taps	6. Seated calf raise and toe-tap
7. Towel wring/wrist curl	7. Tennis ball squeeze
8. Shuttle walks (Fartlek style – varying pace/speed)	8. Shuttle walk – maintain even pace
Optional floor-based MSE stations	*Alternative seated MSE stations*
1. Back raises/extensions	1. Seated back extension
2. Press-ups	2. Wall press-up
3. Static abdominal contraction lying	3. Static abdominal contraction – seated
4. Pelvic floor (standing)	4. Seated pelvic floor

NB: floor-based exercises are only recommended for those persons who can comfortably get up and down from the floor.

NB: You can swap station 5 with station 3 to reduce amount of consecutive leg work if desired.

Table 14.8	General warm-down for active older adults	
Timing	**Exercise/activity**	**Purpose**
1 min 30 secs	Brisk walk in a circle, reducing pace progressively. Walk into space facing one side of hall/room	Maintain intensity of circuit
1 min 30 secs	Gentle side squats right (6.9). March in place, repeat left, progressively lowering intensity	Lowering intensity
1 min	Gentle walk around in any direction, rolling shoulders (6.1). Move to a wall	Lowering intensity and loosening shoulders
1 min	Calf stretch (7.3) with wall support right and left	Lengthening muscles
1 min	Walk anywhere, then stand in place to stretch latissimus dorsi/pectorals and triceps (7.5/7.18/7.6). Move to wall	Lowering intensity and lengthening muscles
30 secs	Quad stretch right and left, using wall for balance. Use towel around ankle, or perform small range of motion hip flexor stretch (7.15) as alternatives	Lengthening muscles
1 min	Seated on floor or chair – back of thigh stretch (7.14, seated)	
1 min	Seated on floor or chair – inner thigh stretch (7.13,)	
1 min 30 secs	Come to standing and gently walk anywhere, rolling shoulders	Revitalise
Total time – 10 mins		

Fig 14.1 Circuit One

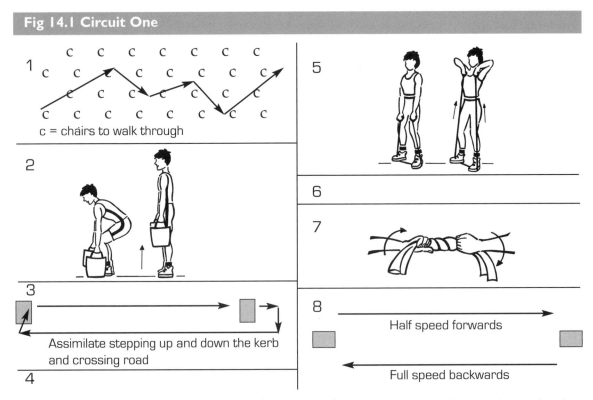

c = chairs to walk through

Circuit One: 1. Walk through crowds; 2. Dead lift (shopping bags); 3. Cross the road; 4. Shoulder press; 5. Standing upright row with resistance bands; 6. Calf raise x 5/Toe raise x 5 then repeat; 7. Towel wring 8. Shuttle walk. NB: Can swap station 5 with station 3 to reduce amount of consecutive legwork if desired.

General circuit training for the chair-bound older adult

Circuit Two

- Six to eight stations, the emphasis being on functional benefit (i.e. comb hair, pelvic floor)
- The aim should be to encourage some activity and mobility movement and have fun. Fitness improvements will be somewhat limited for this population. Ensure movements are performed with control, at a slower pace
- Work ratio: 20–30 secs
- Rest ratio: 10–15 secs, while explaining the next exercise. Participants could be encouraged to clap hands as a rest. Alternatively, a sponge ball could be passed around in a circle from one participant to another in-between exercises. This would suffice as a rest, will add some fun and requires co-ordination skills. Allow time for transition between movements
- Command-style circuit in that everyone performs the same exercise together. Arrange seats in a circular format
- Music can be used to make for a more social environment
- Teaching to ensure correct technique and controlled movements should be the emphasis
- Total time = 10 mins approximately.

Table 14.9	General warm-up for chair-bound older adults	
Timing	**Exercise/activity**	**Purpose**
30 secs	Seated shoulder lifts and shoulder rolls (6.1)	Shoulder mobility
I min	Arm sways side to side, then forwards and backwards	Pulse-raising
30 secs	Point and flex feet	Ankle mobility
30 secs	Seated marching	Pulse-raising
30 secs	Knee lifts (6.6)	Hip mobility and pulse-raising
I min	Finger touches and wrist circles	Finger and wrist mobility
4 mins	Repeat all of the above with larger range of motion	As above
30 secs	Side twists (6.3)	Spine mobility
30 secs	Side bends (6.2)	
30 secs	Seated marching and swinging arms	General pulse-raising
30 secs	Seated step and tap with biceps curls	Elbow mobility and pulse-raising
2 mins	Repeat above (from side twists)	General pulse-raising
Total time – 12 mins		
2 mins	Stretch latissimus dorsi/pectorals and triceps (7.5/7.18/7.6) with gentle shoulder mobility in-between	Lengthening muscles
2 mins	Heel digs moving into seated back of thigh stretch (7.14) right and left	
2 mins	Wiggle around to left side of chair, balancing carefully, extending right leg into hip flexor (7.15) and quadriceps stretch; repeat left	
Total time for stretching – 6 mins **Total time for warm-up – 18 mins**		

Table 14.10	Circuit Two	
Exercise stations	**Alternatives**
1. Getting out of the chair	1. Leg extensions
2. Shoulder press	2. Lateral raise
3. Static abdominal contraction	3. Pelvic floor squeeze
4. Seated calf raise	4. Point and flex the ankle
5. Seated – marching legs	5. Leg slides/extensions
6. Combing hair	–
7. Step taps	7. Toe taps
8. Triceps kickbacks	–

NB: it is recommended that some specific exercises to target the pelvic floor muscles are also included.

Pelvic floor

This exercise can be performed whilst lying, seated or standing:
- Tighten the ring of muscles around the anus. Pull the muscles of the vagina inwards and upwards, and at the same time squeeze the muscles around the front passage (urethra).
- Hold the contraction for a few secs, release and repeat.
- Breathe comfortably throughout. Work towards breathing out as the muscles contract and breathing in as they relax.

NB: please refer to *The Complete Guide to Postnatal Fitness*, Judy DiFiore (A&C Black) for more information on the pelvic floor muscles.

Table 14.11	General warm-down for chair-bound older adults	
Timing	**Exercise/activity**	**Purpose**
30 secs	Seated shoulder lifts and shoulder rolls (6.1)	Shoulder mobility
30 secs	Chest stretch (7.7) and triceps (7.6) – seated	Maintenance stretching
1 min	Arm sways side to side, then forwards and backwards	Pulse-raising
30 secs	Stretch latissimus dorsi and obliques (7.5/7.9)	Maintenance stretching
30 secs	Seated marching	Pulse-raising
1 min	Finger touches and wrist circles	Finger and wrist mobility
1 min	Ankle circles	Ankle mobility
30 secs	Seated marching and swinging arms	General pulse-raising
2 mins	Heel digs moving into seated back of thigh stretch (7.14) right and left	Lengthening muscles
2 mins	Wiggle around to left side of chair, balancing carefully, extending right leg into hip flexor (7.15) and quadriceps stretch; repeat left	
Total warm-down time – 9.5 mins **Finish session with some social interaction, e.g. tea/biscuits and a chat**		

NB: pulse-raising moves are included to maintain body temperature, add variety and assist with keeping the body mobile throughout the component.

OUTDOOR CIRCUITS OR FITNESS TRAILS

15

What are the benefits of outdoor fitness trails?

With the change of the seasons experienced in most countries there is absolutely no need to restrict workouts to the gym environment. The aim of the fitness trail is to encourage those people who do not normally participate in gym activities but who enjoy the great outdoors to incorporate some basic circuit training exercises into their daily or weekly activities. The trail also affords the opportunity for a more intense form of physical conditioning for those already at a reasonable level of fitness.

The fitness trail concept was developed in Scandinavia, Germany and Switzerland. In recent years the concept has been widely adopted in the UK, but not to its fullest potential. There remains a belief that you have to be a member of a gym and use its many high-tech pieces of cardiovascular and resistance-training equipment in order to achieve fitness gains. The reality is that our bodies can be exercised just as effectively without complex machines. Using our own body weight in conjunction with the natural terrain (e.g. logs, steps, seats, slopes, etc.) can help us achieve the desired whole body muscular strength and endurance, and cardiovascular workouts outlined in Chapter 9 at virtually no cost at all. Circuit training is ideally suited to the outdoor environment, be it park, river path, sea front or simply your local neighbourhood.

A circuit can be performed by running, jogging or walking for a set period of time, then stopping and performing an exercise that works a specific muscle or muscle group using body weight in conjunction with the available resources (benches, steps, etc.). A repetition range of between 8–12 reps is sufficient, provided the target muscles have been challenged, then running or walking to the next station can be resumed. The inclusion of rubber resistance bands can greatly increase both the choice and intensity of the exercises performed.

Intensity and duration can be varied in the following ways:

- by increasing or decreasing the intensity of the walk/run/jog between stations
- by increasing or decreasing the time of the walk/run between the exercise stations
- by alternating between running and walking to reach each station
- by selecting a steep or flat terrain according to intensity required.

How to plan a fitness trail

There is no specific layout for a fitness trail, although a permanent course of manufactured stations can be placed around a park, forest or sea front. Examples of such trails are given in Figure 15.1. Various distances from 400 m to 5,000 m can be marked. To plan a trail for your class all that is required is a map of the area, a pedometer and some tracing paper. Once a location has been identified on the map, walk the whole course to ensure that it is suitable and to check the distance from start to finish. Repeat the walk and look for suitable sites for the placement of exercise stations. You may want to take the following factors into consideration when looking for exercise station placements:

- example 1 (bench – can be used for triceps dips)
- example 2 (monkey bars – used for hand walk or pull-ups)
- example 3 (flat ground for sit-ups)
- example 4 (hills – for uphill walks/runs).

It is also important to ensure that any site chosen as an exercise station is a permanent structure, on stable ground and with good drainage. Also note any inclines and/or detours for increased/reduced resistance.

As you walk around the course use the tracing paper as an overlay on the map to make notes. Once the planning is complete use the overlaid drawing to produce a route map (see Figure 15.1).

Fig 15.1 Outdoor circuit

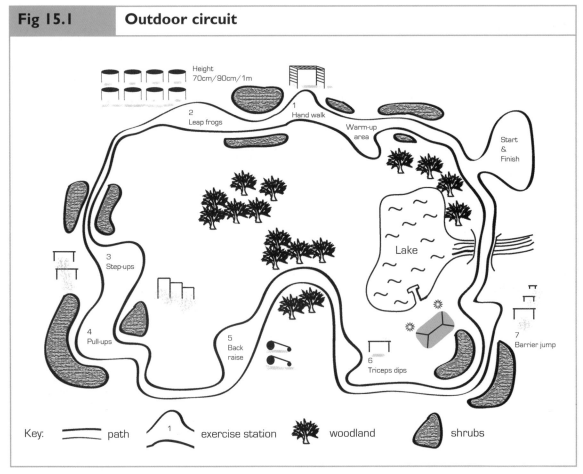

Directions and instructions regarding the fitness trails can be put on notice boards or handed out to participants on paper. In addition there should be notice boards at each exercise station, explaining the exercise to be performed in both words and pictures. The information required on the board is shown in Figure 15.2 and should include:

• Diagram of exercises
• Coaching Points
• Repetitions
• Other fitness trail information.

The stations can be strategically placed around the trail and made of wood or metal. If planning permission for the construction of a permanent trail is not forthcoming, don't worry – familiarity with your local park or woodland and a creative flair for designing exercises will give you a fitness trail that can be adapted to suit the needs of your class without leaving a permanent scar on the environment.

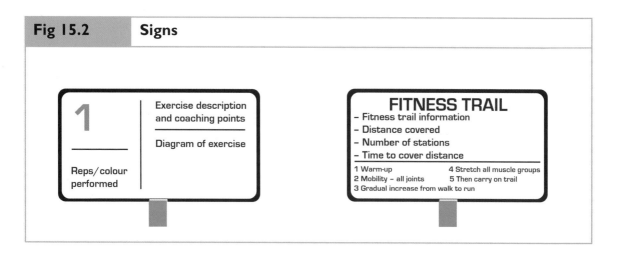

Fig 15.2   **Signs**

Table 15.1	Example outdoor circuit session

Part of circuit	Description
Warm-up – time?	Walk at a comfortable pace for about 5 mins, during which mobility of all major joints is carried out (ankles, knees, hips, spine, shoulder, elbows). Continue to walk at this pace for a further 5 mins, stopping periodically to perform a series of stretching exercises (see Chapter 7) (calves, anterior tibialis, hamstrings, quads, adductors, abductors, glutes, hip flexors, erector spinae, pectorals, traps, deltoids, triceps). The upper body can be stretched while still walking, provided the class is skilled enough to maintain correct posture and technique
Main circuit – time?	Continue to walk, only this time at an increased pace of 3 mph or at a brisk walk for the next 5 mins. Stop and carry out 10 repetitions of a lunge (alternate legs leading). Increase the pace to either a jog or a quicker walking pace for another 5 mins, then stop and perform 10 repetitions of a power squat. Quick walk or run for the next 5 mins, then stop and carry out tuck jumps for 10 repetitions. Quick walking/running for the next 5 mins, then stop and perform jumping jacks
Cool-down – time?	Walk/run for 5 mins, gradually decreasing the pace of the walk/run, then perform a series of cooling down stretches (chest, back and arms). Continue to walk at a slower pace, then stop and carry out lower body stretches using the natural terrain, e.g. benches or steps to aid stretching calves, hip flexors, hamstrings, quadriceps, gluteals, adductors and abductors.

Total warm-down time – 40 mins

Upper body exercises can be included if desired during the stops. Walk/running times can be increased or decreased.

Walking techniques

The different walking techniques listed can be used in isolation or combined together to provide an interval approach to the outdoor walking circuit workout. One of the greatest aspects of fitness walking is its simplicity – it can be performed by a range of groups. Muscular strength and endurance activities can also be included to provide a more balanced workout.

The advantages of using a variety of walking techniques throughout the workout include the following:

- adds variety and jazzes up the walking
- keeps individuals challenged
- assists motivation.

The following points on technique will make participants' walking more effective, enjoyable and safer. Instructors should resist the temptation to take this inherently simple, pleasurable activity and make it too complicated.

Walking for Health (Level 1)

Head

The head should be held in a neutral position and centred to be in line with the spine. The chin should be parallel to the ground. Focus the eyes without lowering the chin.

Shoulders

The shoulders should be pulled back and down in a relaxed position rather than rounded. Tightness in the shoulders can impair arm swing.

Chest

The chest should be lifted to help maintain spinal alignment.

Abdominals

Transversus abdominis muscle should be contracted throughout the walk to maintain a neutral spine.

Arm Action

The arm swing should be natural and comfortable with elbows relaxed as the arms swing in opposition to the legs. Arms should swing close to the side of the body and not across the front of the body.

Leg Action

The stride length should be comfortable and will vary from one individual to another.

Foot Placement

The heel should land first, with a rolling through to the toes (foot rolls from heel to toes).

Fitness Walking (Level 2)

Posture (see specific guidelines for Level 1)

Keep head up, chin parallel to the floor, eyes looking forwards, shoulders back, down and relaxed, and chest lifted. Abdominals should be contracted lightly, maintaining a neutral spine position.

Arm Action

The arms should be bent to approximately 90 degrees at the elbow joint (giving a shorter length pendulum which will produce a faster arm swing). A quicker arm swing causes an increase in leg speed. The movement of the arms is produced at the shoulder and not from the elbow. Arms should swing forwards and backwards and not across the centre line of the body. Hands should be held in a loose fist. The arms naturally swing in opposition to the legs.

Leg Action

The knee of the right leg should be almost fully extended when the right foot is planted on the ground (but not hyper-extended).

Hip Action

The pelvis will have a slight rotation. As walking speed increases, so will this rotation. This should be a natural biomechanical movement.

Foot Placement

As the heel is planted on the ground the toes are raised towards the shins (dorsiflexion). The foot then rolls from heel to toe under control with a final push off from the ball of the foot.

Forward Lean

There is a definite forward lean from the ankles and not the hips. (Achieve a feeling of 'falling forwards' into each step.)

Race Walking (Level 3)

Posture (see specific guidelines listed at Level 1)

Keep the head up, chin parallel to the floor, eyes looking forwards, shoulders back, down and relaxed, and chest lifted. Abdominals should be contracted to maintain a neutral spine.

Arm Action

The elbows are bent at approximately 90 degrees (same as for fitness walking). However, as the arms swing forwards, they should cross closer to the centre of the body and swing no higher than the sternum. The walker should consciously drive the elbows back and keep them close to the body. A quicker arm swing will increase leg speed.

Leg Action

The legs need to be pulled forwards more quickly. Concentration should be on increasing stride frequency, not stride length. As the right leg swings forwards, the supporting or left leg should remain straight.

Hip Action

Hip rotation plays a crucial role in race walking. The pelvis moves or rotates forwards and backwards with a minimum of side-to-side motion. As the hip of the advancing leg reaches maximum forward rotation, the hip drops or tilts down.

Foot Placement

Walkers should keep the ball of the rear foot on the ground until the heel of the forward leg has contact with the ground. As the heel of the advancing leg contacts the ground, its ankle should be dorsiflexed to about 90 degrees. Walking at these higher speeds means the foot should form a continuous straight line, with the inner edge of one foot landing in line with the inner edge of the other foot (like walking on a tightrope).

Forward Lean

Walkers should have a slight forward lean from the ankles (*not* the hips).

Other walking activities

The following walking activities can be used at intervals in a walking programme to change the intensity, add variety and continue the challenge of the walking circuit.

There and Back

Walk forwards to a designated landmark. When the landmark has been reached, turn around and walk back to the trainer. A walking pace above baseline pace should be used, dependent on fitness level.

Send Them Back

Walk back to a designated landmark already passed, then catch up. A walking pace above baseline should be used, dependent on fitness level.

NB: both the above activities can be used when the trainer maintains the baseline pace whilst moving forwards.

Taking Shortcuts

The trainer walks along a designated route/path while sending walkers on a much longer route. The two routes should meet and so should the walkers.

First Past the Post

The trainer sends the walkers off to a landmark away in the distance. Walkers use a pace they can sustain above baseline. Once the first person has reached the landmark, all walkers, wherever they are, turn around and walk back to the starting point. First past the post should also be the first to finish.

Hare and Hounds

Send slower walkers off at set timed intervals. The quicker walkers have to catch the slower walkers up.

NB: the above walking activities are ideal when working with either groups with a mixed fitness level or one-on-one.

Outdoor Walking Circuit Workout Plan

The three levels of walking described can be manipulated within a session and used to provide an interval training approach of higher and lower speeds (pace). In addition, some body weight exercises can be incorporated to provide muscular strength and endurance work within the programme. An effective walking workout can be achieved for all levels of fitness.

Table 15.2	Walking circuit with cardiovascular focus
Warm up	**10 mins**
Pulse-raising and mobility	5 mins Using Level 1 technique, gradually increase the pace, incorporate mobility of the joints early in the warm-up
Stretching	2 mins Stretch muscles to be used in main workout as appropriate
Re-warm and build intensity	3 mins Gradually increase the pace and change the technique to Level 2 to find a sustainable pace, which will be the baseline for the workout.
Main workout	**20 mins**
Walking circuit	1 min Lunge walking – continuous lunging using alternative lead leg, taking a slight pause in between when both feet are together. (Gradually build up to 1 minute) 1 min Fast walking pace – increase pace of walking above baseline pace 1 min Slow down to baseline pace, or just below, to achieve heart rate recovery 1 min Sprint walk intervals – choose a selection of objects (trees, benches, waste bins or similar) in the distance. Walk as fast as you can (Level 2 / Level 3 technique) to that object; reduce walk intensity to recover then repeat for the full minute 3 mins Slow pace down to baseline speed / technique, to recover from sprint intervals 1 min Press-ups, tree press-ups or bench dips – whichever is preferred and sustainable for 1 minute. (Over sessions, time can gradually be built up from 30 secs to the minute) 1 min Spotty dogs – scissor/split jumps, either legs only while leaning against a tree, or full spotty dogs. (Over sessions, time can gradually be built up from 30 secs to the minute) 1 min Speed Walk – increase your speed and change to the appropriate technique so that you feel you are walking hard. (Can start with 2 separate 30-second speed walks with a short recovery between and work up to the minute)

Table 15.2	Walking circuit with cardiovascular focus cont.
	3 mins Slow pace down to baseline speed / technique, to recover from the speed walk
	1 min Long jumps – find a relatively flat area and begin with feet together. Lower into a slight squat and jump forwards with both feet as far as you can, swinging your arms to help propel you forwards. Continue leaping forward for 30 secs, take a walking break, and then continue for another 30 secs. (Due to the high intensity of this activity four sections of 15 secs separated by a walking recovery can be a starting point)
	1 min Speed walk – walk at a relatively quick pace to reduce heart rate and intensity a touch
	1 min High knee lifts – walk or jog for a minute, during which aim to get your knees level with your hips
	1 min Low knee – walk or jog for a minute, during which bring heels to bottom
	3 mins Walk or jog – slow down to baseline.
Cool-down	**5 mins**
Pulse-lowering	3 mins Gradually reduce pace, moving through the levels to a low Level 1
Stretch	2 mins Stretch all muscles worked through main workout Focus on lower body.

Walking for seniors and beginners

When planning a walking session for the above target groups/individuals, the following may help.

Separate the session into three sections, the first lasting 5 mins. Walking during this time can be at a stroll (acts as a warm-up). The second 5 mins (or proportion of this, dependent on walkers' fitness/ability) should be walked at a much quicker pace to invoke a quicker heart and breathing rate. Correct walking technique should be introduced and reinforced throughout this time. The last 5 mins will act as the cool-down, and again can be performed at a strolling pace.

This should be repeated two to three times in the first few weeks. Adding an additional 2–3 mins to the middle section each week until 30 mins can be completed on most days of the week (which falls in line with the Department of Health guidelines, 2005). Warm-up and cool-down times can be adjusted accordingly.

If monitoring the intensity of walking via heart rate or RPE then it should be kept between 50 and 69 per cent MHR or 2–4 RPE (scale 1–10), during the workout phase of the walk. Walking should be performed on a flat route initially, with small inclines added at a later date, as long as this does not increase the physical stress on the walkers.

How can I check what speed am I walking?

The following is a way of estimating pace judgment, but is only a guide.

110–120 steps per minute = 3.0mph
(40 steps in 20 secs)

124–135 steps per minute = 4.0mph
(45 steps in 20 secs)

145–155 steps per minute = 5.0mph
(50 steps in 20 secs)

Grading walkers' ability

The following is just a guide (from Sonning Common Health Walks, see www.healthwalks. freeserve.co.uk) to help match walkers' fitness and ability to the correct walking programme intensity and route:

Level A walkers – walk at over 4.0 mph and do not find hills a major problem.

Level B walkers – walk at between 3.5 and 4.0 mph on the flat, but tend to find hills a struggle.

Level C walkers – walk below 3.0 mph and find everything a struggle.

Walk/run workouts

Complete a 10-min warm-up, including stretching, using a health walking technique, gradually increasing the pace throughout the 10 mins until the pace warrants a fitness walking technique. Continue to walk at this pace until an RPE of 5/6 is reached. The workout can now start (see Table 15.3).

Table 15.3	Walk/run workout		
Mode	RPE	HR	Time
Walking	5-6	70-80%	2 mins
Running	6-7	75-85%	2 mins
Walking	5-6	70-80%	3 mins
Running	6-7	75-85%	3 mins
Walking	5-6	70-80%	3 mins
Running	6-7	75-85%	3 mins
Walking	5-6	70-80%	2 mins
Running	6-7	75-85%	2 mins
Walking	4-5	60-70%	2 mins

Cool down, further decreasing the pace to a health walking technique for a further 3–5 mins. Finish the session with a stretch of the targeted muscle groups.

SPORT-SPECIFIC CIRCUIT TRAINING

16

Sportspeople are always at risk of over-training and building up the intensity of their programmes too quickly. The occurrence of repetitive strain and overuse injuries is common. Training or cross-training can improve and maintain physical fitness and assist with the development of specific skills.

This chapter explores the benefits of circuit training specifically for the sportsperson. It also outlines an appropriate session structure, and provides guidelines for designing a variety of sport-specific circuits.

What are the benefits of circuit training for the sportsperson?

The sportsperson may use circuit training within a general conditioning programme. Alternatively, they may use circuit training to develop specific skills. Sports coaches usually plan a season of activities for the athlete or sportsperson. This is known as periodisation. The aims and goals at each stage of seasonal training will vary slightly according to the needs of the sport and the individual sportsperson. A simple method of breaking down seasonal training regimes is as follows:

- pre-season training or cross-training
- main season cross-training
- post-season training or cross-training
- injury rehabilitation.

Pre-season

The primary aim of pre-season training is to develop a base level of fitness in all components of physical fitness. These include muscular strength and endurance, cardiovascular fitness and flexibility. Once a base level of fitness is achieved, the sportsperson can then work towards developing the specific skills that will enhance their performance in their chosen sporting event. These will vary depending on the sporting activity, but may include one or more of the following: power, speed, balance, agility, co-ordination, etc. Guidelines for improving fitness in each of these components are discussed in Chapter 1.

Main season

During main season training, the sportsperson will need to develop and enhance their sport-specific skills further. They will also need to maintain their existing fitness level. Cross-training using circuits will lessen the risk of injury when training to improve these skills.

Post-season

The primary aim of post-season training is to provide an active recovery period for the body. The body will need time to recuperate and recover from the stresses placed upon it from competitive activity. The programme of activities provided at this stage should be sufficient to maintain a reasonable level of physical fitness. However, they should be less demanding. A greater emphasis can be placed on mobility and stretching activities.

Injury rehabilitation

Injury can leave the sportsperson feeling frustrated and desperate to get back to training in order to restore their fitness level. It is essential that the initial rehabilitation work prescribed by a physiotherapist is completed before normal training resumes. Furthermore, when returning to exercise, the programme should be built up gradually and with guidance from the physiotherapist. Readers should refer to other specific texts and take further training to deal with injury rehabilitation work.

How should the sport-specific training session be structured?

Sport-specific training should follow the same session structure as any other. The session should be preceded by an adequate period of warming up and concluded with an adequate period of cooling down. The design of the main session will be dependent on the athlete's reasons for participating. It is wise to include activities to improve all components of physical fitness. However, specific attention may need to be given to:

* replicating the activities performed maximally throughout the sport
* counter-balancing the strength of the opposing muscles to those used maximally throughout the activity
* developing flexibility in muscles that are required to lengthen quickly while their opposing muscle is contracting forcefully

(e.g. to kick a ball, the quadriceps contract forcefully. Their opposing muscle group, the hamstrings, needs to be sufficiently flexible to relax and lengthen. If it is not, there is a greater risk of the muscle tearing). An appropriate session structure is outlined in Table 16.1.

How to analyse needs for effective sport-specific circuit training programmes

To design an effective sport-specific training session, it is necessary to conduct a needs analysis for the specific sport. Each of the following needs to be considered:

* the main movement activities and skills used in the sport
* how the joints move
* which muscles are involved and how they contract (concentric, eccentric, isometric and plyometric)
* predominant energy pathway used (aerobic/anaerobic)
* common injuries associated with a particular sport.

Spending time on this analysis will ensure that the circuit designed will be safe, effective and follow the principles of specificity. Observing a video recording of a sporting activity will also allow one to analyse and break down the movements more specifically. Once the main activities have been identified, it is necessary to identify ways of replicating these movements.

Needs analysis assessments for specific sports, with example lesson plans, are provided at the end of this chapter.

Table 16.1	Structuring a sport-specific circuit
Warm-up component	• mobility and pulse-raising – target joints used throughout the main workout • preparatory stretches – include extra static or range of motion stretches for muscles which will need to move through an extended range of motion during the main workout • re-warm specific to the main activity. Could be a small-sided controlled team game performed at lower intensity, the aim being to rehearse skills rather than boost intensity too much.
Main workout	• include activities to train cardiovascular fitness • include activities to replicate activities of the specific sport (skill, power, etc.) • include activities to strengthen opposing muscle groups to counter-balance and compensate for overuse in sporting activities.
Cool-down	• cooling down activities to lower heart rate and assist with the removal of waste products that affect the metabolism of the muscle physiology. Activities should be specific to the main activity • stretch all muscles worked • develop less flexible muscles

Table 16.2 is a very simple breakdown of two of the main movements required when playing football. However, even this basic analysis provides evidence that the quadriceps muscles receive a greater amount of work than their antagonist, the hamstrings. The following activities should therefore be considered:

• strengthening work for the quadriceps and hip flexors as the main prime movers
• counterbalancing strengthening work for the hamstrings
• flexibility work for the hamstrings and gluteals to ensure these muscles have sufficient range of motion to lengthen when their opposing muscles contract so forcefully
• flexibility work for all muscles that are contracting strongly throughout the activity, i.e. quadriceps, gastrocnemius, soleus, erector spinae, to maintain flexibility
• improvement of cardiovascular fitness

• improvement of anaerobic fitness – explosive bursts.

Further consideration, specifically in team sports, would need to be given to the position in which the sportsperson plays. Sports coaches are advised to seek information from other specific sporting texts and up-to-date research to assist their planning for position-specific circuit training.

Table 16.2	Breakdown of the joint actions and muscles working for two of the main activities in football		
Movement	Joint action	Prime mover (muscle that contracts to bring about the movement)	Antagonist (muscle that lengthens when prime mover contracts)
Kicking	Hip flexion	Hip flexor, quadriceps	Gluteals, hamstrings
Kicking	Knee extension	Quadriceps	Hamstrings
Running	Hip flexion	Hip flexor, quadriceps	Gluteals, hamstrings
Running	Hip extension	Gluteals, hamstrings	Hip flexor, quadriceps
Running	Ankle dorsiflexion	Tibialis anterior	Gastrocnemius, soleus
Running	Ankle plantarflexion	Gastrocnemius, soleus	Tibialis anterior
Running	Knee extension	Quadriceps	Hamstrings

Lesson plans for specific sports

As we have seen, circuit training can be adapted to suit different fitness and skill levels. The following lesson plans are tailored to specific sporting disciplines. Exercise stations mirror movements and skills used in different sports, and also address the fitness requirements. The timing of each station in the circuit depends on the total time available. The recommendation of 45 secs to 1 minute at each station can be extended. Within the timeframe the aim is to achieve 'overload'. The timeframe will also depend on whether the circuit is 'stand alone' or part of a training schedule.

Athletics

Needs analysis

The general conditioning circuit is not designed for any specific event, but rather to help develop muscular strength, muscular endurance and power. Anaerobic conditioning is particularly important for the athlete, to help an individual tolerate the build-up of lactic acid while performing athletic-specific muscle and joint actions continuously. The need for postural stability has also been accounted for.

Warm-up

The warm-up can be carried out as described in Chapter 6, using the exercises described in Chapter 7. In addition, the pulse-raising component can be achieved by the group using the track (or outdoor area), completing several circuits at different paces, during which upper and lower body stretches can be performed, as described in Chapter 7.

Cool-down

The track (or outside area) can be utilised, with the pace being varied to gain a warming/cooling effect to aid removal of waste products (lactic acid) and prepare the body for the main part of the stretch. Development of range of movement should be carried out indoors, where possible, to aid muscle warmth retention and comfort.

Specific muscles used: iliopsoas; quadriceps; hamstrings; gluteals; calves; pectoralis; latissimus dorsi; deltoids.

Joints used: Hips; knees; ankles; shoulders.

Predominant energy pathway: aerobic/anaerobic (dependent on event).

Flexibility focus: calves; iliopsoas.

Equipment required: gym benches/step boxes; various strength resistance bands; sets of 1–2 kg dumbbells; gym mats; gym (stability) balls; suitable wall.

Table 16.3	Athletics circuit
Station 1	**Arm driving** Emphasis: muscle endurance (anterior & posterior deltoid) Stand in a stable position, one foot in front of the other, maintaining good core spine stability. Keeping arms close to the body and bent at the elbows, swing arms backwards and forwards from the shoulders. The action of the arm swing must be continuous for the given time frame. Athletes can adopt various levels of forward lean throughout the exercise, but it is important to work on maintaining a stable trunk position. Equipment: 1–2 kg dumbbells
Station 2	**Alternate leg steps** Emphasis: muscle strength/explosive power (gastrocnemius, quadriceps, gluteus maximus) Stand with one foot on a bench approximately 50 cm high. Drive up off that one leg to achieve full extension, change legs on the way down, and then repeat the exercise with the other leg. Carry on doing this without the use of the arms for the given time frame. Avoid hyperextension of the knee joint at the end of the range of movement. Equipment: Step benches

Table 16.3	Athletics circuit cont.

Station 3	**Knee pick-up** Emphasis: muscle strength/endurance (hip flexor) Stand an arm's distance away from a wall, hands supporting the body, with elbows slightly bent. Lean forwards and carry out the running action with emphasis on the knee pick-up. Ankle weights can be used for added resistance. Equipment: Supporting wall
Station 4	**Back extension** Emphasis: muscle endurance (erector spinae group) Lie face down (prone) on the floor or on top of either a stability 'gym' ball or the end of a gym bench/step box, supported from the waist down. Raise the trunk up as far as is comfortable without excessive hyperextension and lower back to the start position. This exercise must be done using a slow, controlled action. For added resistance a medicine ball or dumbbell can be used. Equipment: Gym ball/step benches
Station 5	**Abdominal work** All abdominal muscles should be exercised to achieve full stability of a vulnerable area of the body. The following exercises are recommended: **Curl-up** Emphasis: muscle endurance (rectus abdominis, interior & exterior obliques) Lie on the floor, on your back (supine), knees bent and feet flat on the floor. The arms can be placed in a position suitable to the fitness level of the athlete, but avoid grabbing behind the head. Pull the 'abs' in tight and curl the spine towards the knees. Be sure to leave a gap between the chin and the chest. Lower under control using a slow speed until the shoulders touch the floor then repeat. This exercise can be carried out in a similar way using a stability 'gym' ball. Equipment: Gym ball **The Plank** Emphasis: muscle endurance (transversus abdominis) Lie face down on a mat with the forehead supported on the back of the hands. The chest, hips, knees and feet must be supported on the floor. Relax the whole body, breathe in while maintaining this relaxed body position, then breathe out. Pull the belly button (umbilicus) in tight towards the spine and hold this position. Maintain a breathing rhythm and keep the body relaxed. Hold for as long as possible. Repeat. Equipment: Mat

Table 16.3	Athletics circuit cont.
Station 6	**Single leg bounding** Emphasis: muscle strength/power (gastrocnemius, quadriceps, gluteus maximus, hamstrings, hip flexors) (Jumps using single leg take off, bringing knee up to hip height.) To start this exercise aim to achieve a slight lean forwards. Just as the body starts to lose balance, lift the knee and drive off the supporting leg, achieving full extension through the ankle joint. Start off walking then progress to running.
Station 7	**Leg curls** Emphasis: muscle strength/endurance (hamstrings) Lie face down (prone) on top of a bench or on the floor, close to an anchor point on a wall. Tie an exercise rubber tube to the anchor point, with the other end tied around the ankles of the athlete. Maintaining good stability of the upper body, curl the lower leg towards the body and return to the start position under control. This exercise can be performed either using both legs together or single legs alternately. Equipment: Resistance rubber band
Station 8	**Lunge walking** Emphasis: muscular endurance (quadriceps, gluteals, hamstring) Stand with feet hip-width apart, take an extended step forwards and bend the front knee, keeping the knee behind the toes. The rear leg should be close to full extension. Keep the upper body in an upright position with 'abs' tight, and then repeat the exercise using the other leg for the given time frame.
Station 9	**Squat with calf raises** Emphasis: muscle strength (gastrocnemius, quadriceps, gluteus maximus, hamstrings) Stand with feet hip-width apart, feet facing forwards. During the lowering phase, bend at the hips and knees, keeping the knees in line with the feet and behind the toes. At the bottom of the squat the hips should be above the knees. Try to keep the upper body in as upright a position as possible; there may be a natural slight lean forwards. When rising, lead with the shoulders and stand up, following the movement up onto the toes. This exercise can be done using either both legs together or single legs. When using single legs, use the arms to mimic the running act to aid balance. The whole action should be continuous and dynamic.
Station 10	**Bench hopping** Emphasis: muscle strength/power (gastrocnemius, quadriceps, gluteals); anaerobic conditioning, muscle endurance (hip flexors)

Table 16.3	Athletics circuit cont.
	Stand facing a line of benches and perform a single-legged take-off to clear the bench, landing on the other leg, being sure to bend the knee to absorb the impact. Now take off using the other leg and clear the bench again. Repeat this action all the way down the length of the bench. To get back to the start, jog using a very fast knee pick-up with very slow forward movement, then repeat the bench jumps again.
	Equipment: Six step benches

Badminton

Needs analysis

The game requires the players to be able to bend, stretch and reach to the left, right and overhead of their playing position. They need to be very agile about the court, to attack and defend shots both high and low, and to the front and back of the court. This circuit has been designed with these needs in mind.

Warm-up

A general type of warm-up can be performed to achieve the desired effect prior to starting the badminton circuit, providing the guidelines in Chapters 6 and 7 have been followed. Suggest players carry out their exercises with racket in hand. Further pulse-raising can be achieved by carrying out a controlled 'knock-up' to each other, varying the shot and pace of shot.

Cool-down

Whole body stretching as described in Chapter 7 with the emphasis on those muscle groups in the flexibility focus.

Specific muscles used: calves; quadriceps; gluteals; pectoralis; triceps; brachioradialis; deltoids.

Joints used: hips; knees; ankles; shoulders; wrists; elbows.

Specific muscle action: isotonic – above muscles; isometric – postural muscles of the trunk (abs; erector spinae).

Predominant energy pathway: aerobic.

Flexibility focus: triceps; wrist flexors and extensors; hip flexors; calves; hamstrings.

Equipment required: Badminton racket for each player; shuttlecocks; posts and nets; marked-out court; mats; resistance bands; marker cones; short metal/wooden bar; length of cordage; 2.5–5 kg plates.

Table 16.4	Badminton Circuit
Station 1	**Retrieve and smash** Emphasis: anaerobic conditioning, skill, muscle endurance (gastrocnemius, quadriceps, gluteals, deltoids, triceps) Run forward 6 ft, touch the floor with the racket head or hand, close to the feet, then run backwards to the back of the court, jump and smash. If possible, hit a ball/shuttle suspended from above or mimic hitting a shuttle. Repeat. Equipment: Badminton racket, shuttlecock
Station 2	**Traverse the net** Emphasis: anaerobic conditioning, muscular endurance (hamstring, quadriceps, adductors, gluteals) Start in the centre of the court, side step to a cone, do a side lunge with an outstretched arm, and reach and touch the floor with the racket head. Repeat to the opposite side of the court: side lunge, reach and touch the floor on the backhand side. Repeat. Equipment: Two marking cones, badminton racket
Station 3	**Tour of half court** Emphasis: anaerobic conditioning, skill Using half the court, place four cones at each corner. Facing the net at all times, run around the cones. When the player reaches the net they should retrieve a drop shot by reaching down and touching the floor with the racket head, side step across court making sure not to cross over legs, jump and smash a suspended shuttle/ball or just simulate the action, run backwards to the back court line and reach backwards on the forehand side to touch the floor. Then side step across the court and jump, reach up and simulate a backhand smash or hit a suspended shuttle. Repeat. Equipment: Four marker cones, net and posts, badminton racket
Station 4	**Shuffle the shuttle** Emphasis: anaerobic conditioning Have three stations 6 ft apart; at each station place a shuttlecock. Stand behind the line of shuttlecocks at one end. Pick up the first shuttle with the racket hand and run sideways, making sure not to cross the legs, over to the second shuttle. Using only the racket hand, replace the shuttle in hand with the one on the floor. Then run to the end station and do the same. The pick-ups can be forehand or backhand. Equipment: Three shuttlecocks per person

Table 16.4	Badminton Circuit cont.
Station 5	**Attack and defend** Emphasis: anaerobic conditioning, muscle strength/endurance (gastrocnemius, quadriceps, gluteals) From a starting line, run forwards 6 ft, jump and simulate a smash or hit a ball suspended 10–12 ft from the ground. Run backwards 12 ft, reach down, and touch a mark on the floor. Alternate on backhand and forehand side. Equipment: Marker cones and badminton rackets
Station 6	Wrist curls Emphasis: muscle endurance (wrist flexors) Use a bar approximately 45 cm long with a length of rope tied to the middle of it and a weight on the other end. Several bars can be provided with different weights loads. Stand with feet hip-width apart to give stability, take hold of the bar at each end, and curl the wrists to wind the weight up; when the weight has reached the top, reverse the action under control. The exercise can either be performed in several ways – arms outstretched, elbows locked by the side, or a combination of both. An alternative to this exercise for the badminton player is the wrist curl. Sit on a seat/bench holding a barbell with an underhand grip, rest the back of the lower arm on the legs, then just using the wrist joint curl the bar upwards and down under control. Equipment: Several short metal/wooden bars 45 cm long with lengths of cordage tied to them holding 2.5–5 kg weight plates
Station 7	**A mini circuit** Emphasis: muscle endurance (pectoralis major, triceps, anterior deltoid, quadriceps, gluteals, gastrocnemius, hamstrings, rectus abdominis, obliques, erector spinae, rotator cuff group (supraspinatus, infraspinatus, teres minor, subscapularis) To include the following exercises: press-ups; squat jumps; abdominal work; back hyperextensions; rotator cuff exercises. Each exercise in this circuit is to be carried out for 45 secs without rest, going around as many times as possible in the time allowed. Equipment: Gym mats and balls, if available.

Basketball

Needs analysis

Specific skills related to basketball are passing, dribbling and shooting, offensive and defensive plays. To this end the following analysis has been used to design appropriate exercises to meet a player's needs, while not overlooking the fitness requirements.

Warm-up

Mobility activities to be performed on court with ball in hand, covering whole body mobility as described in Chapter 6. Basic dribbling skills can be incorporated to gain a pulse-raising effect. Stretches, with emphasis on calves, hamstrings, hip flexors, chest, back and triceps, as described in Chapter 7. Further warming (pulse-raising) can be achieved by increasing the pace of the dribbling, passing and shooting practices used, or including a small-sided game: 2 v 2, 3 v 3, etc.

Cool-down

Complete the session with a whole body stretch as laid down in Chapter 7, with emphasis on developing hamstrings, adductors and hip flexors.

Specific muscles used: quadriceps; gluteals; hamstrings; calves; deltoids; shoulders.

Joints used: ankles; knees; hips; shoulders; elbows; wrists.

Predominant energy pathway: aerobic – lactic acid (anaerobic).

Flexibility focus: hamstrings; adductors; hip flexors.

Equipment required: basketball for each player; backboards and hoops; mats; marking cones.

Table 16.5	Basketball Circuit
	Duration: Players perform each activity in pairs. Work for 45 secs with a 15-second rest between stations.
Station 1	**The press** Emphasis: anaerobic conditioning, skill Players negotiate through a zigzag course of cones, one attacking, the other defending, and swap roles after each lap. Equipment: Marking cones, basketball
Station 2	**The wall pass** Emphasis: local muscular endurance (pectoralis group, triceps, anterior deltoid, wrist flexors), skill (reaction) Players keep ball in motion (chest passing), against a wall, while rotating behind each other. Player two receives the ball from player one's pass. Equipment: Basketball, gym wall

Table 16.5	Basketball Circuit cont.
Station 3	**Dribble** Emphasis: anaerobic conditioning Players must always face the front throughout this exercise and negotiate an 'X' shape around the four laid out cones. Equipment: Four marking cones, basketball
Station 4	**The rebound shot** Emphasis: local muscle endurance (triceps, deltoid, core), skill One player shoots; the other player must rebound and score even if the shot was successful, twice if unsuccessful. Equipment: Backboard and hoop, basketball
Station 5	**Lunge dribble** Emphasis: local muscle endurance (quadriceps, gluteals, hamstrings), anaerobic conditioning, skill Players 'lunge' walk between the base line and halfway line, bouncing a ball through the legs with each step; forwards one way, backwards on the return. Equipment: Basketballs
Station 6	**Dribble eight** Emphasis: skill Standing figure of eight dribbles through/around legs. Equipment: Basketball
Station 7	**Bouncing abs** Emphasis: local muscle endurance (rectus abdominis, obliques), skill Players perform abdominal exercise (curl-ups) while keeping the ball bouncing. Equipment: Mats, basketball
Station 8	**The lay-up** Emphasis: skill Alternate hand lay-ups. Equipment: Basketball, backboard and hoop

Boxing

Needs analysis

Boxing is an activity that requires the participant to have a high level of tolerance in order to overcome local muscular fatigue, primarily caused by lactic acid build-up (anaerobic). They also need a high level of aerobic conditioning to aid recovery and the development of skills such as speed, reaction, balance, co-ordination and agility, necessary to survive in the ring. The following analysis shows the main areas that have encouraged the circuit design.

Warm-up

A normal warm-up can be applied to this circuit as described in Chapters 6 and 7. Special attention should be given to mobility of the shoulder, elbow and spinal joints. Additional, more specific warming can be achieved by incorporating activities such as non-contact sparring, and bobbing and weaving moves.

Cool-down

On completion of the circuit, a jog out in the open may be of advantage, to help remove waste while helping to re-warm the body for a whole body stretch. Use the exercises as described in Chapter 7 to achieve this.

Specific muscles used: quadriceps; gluteals; hamstrings; calves; abdominals; back; triceps; deltoids.

Joints used: ankles; knees; hips; spine; shoulders; elbows.

Predominant energy pathway: anaerobic; aerobic recovery.

Flexibility focus: pectorals; deltoids; hamstrings; gluteals; calves; triceps.

Equipment required: punch bags; gloves; skipping ropes; mats; numerous sets of 2 kg dumbbells; gym beam or similar; hanging punch bags or gym ropes; pads; gym benches.

Table 16.6	Boxing circuit
Station 1	**Bob and weave** Emphasis: skill, anaerobic conditioning This activity needs ropes or punch bags hanging from the ceiling, reasonably close together (or anything that can be used as a swinging obstacle). The boxer will have to side step in and out of the obstacles. The idea is to get from one end to the other without being touched by the obstacles. This activity is important for footwork while maintaining defensive position. Equipment: Five punch bags or ropes or equivalent
Station 2	**Pad work** Emphasis: muscle endurance (triceps, pectorals, deltoids, latissimus dorsi), skill, anaerobic conditioning For this exercise it is necessary to work with a coach or someone familiar with the various punches. The idea is that, working in a small area, the boxer will throw punches in the given order. The boxer needs to keep on their toes, maintain good defence and expect the unexpected from the coach. Equipment: Gloves, pads, marker cones
Station 3	**Step and punch** Emphasis: local muscular endurance (quadriceps, gluteals, calves, triceps, pectorals, deltoids) The boxer will need a set of dumbbells and a bench to step on. As the boxer steps on to the bench they throw a punch, and the same when they step off. The higher the step, the more legwork required. The faster the boxer steps, the faster the punching action. Equipment: Sets of dumbbells between 2–5 kg, gym benches or step box
Station 4	**Resistance running** Emphasis: aerobic conditioning Run between two marks, where possible 20 m apart. Carry a heavy weight (this weight could be 2 × 10 kg dumbbells or higher, or two car tyres). Continue the laps over the given time period. Equipment: Dumbbells
Station 5	**Bob and slap** Emphasis: local muscular endurance (quadriceps, gluteals, calves, deltoids, triceps, pectorals), skill For this exercise it is necessary to use a beam or similar, suspended so that it is just below shoulder height. The boxer needs to stand facing forwards and squat under the beam,

Table 16.6	Boxing circuit cont.
	coming up on the other side where they should slap the side of the beam. The exercise is then repeated on the other side of the beam. The boxer carries on doing this the length of the beam. Once at the end, the boxer will repeat the action, only this time walking backwards. Care should be taken to avoid hitting the head on the beam. Equipment: Two volleyball posts with string tied between, or gym beam
Station 6	**Hit the bag** Emphasis: local muscular endurance (calves, quadriceps, gluteals, deltoids, triceps, pectorals), anaerobic conditioning Keeping light-footed, move around the punch bag, delivering a combination of different punches. The punch bag can either be held by a coach/helper or be free swinging. Equipment: Suspended punch bag, gloves or mits
Station 7	**Mini-circuit** Emphasis: aerobic conditioning, local muscular endurance (abdominal region, erector spinae, deltoids), anaerobic conditioning This can be performed as a station or a separate circuit training session. The circuit should include the following exercises: 1. Skipping – using own style, but keeping feet close to the ground. 2. Full press-ups with a clap – should this exercise be too intense, then revert to a normal press-up, making sure that the arms are one and a half times shoulder-width apart, fingers facing forwards, arms bent, elbows going outwards. Make sure that when arms are at full extension there is a slight bend at the elbow. 3. Sit-ups – using a medicine ball held above the head, sit up until you can touch the wall with the ball. Make sure that the transverse abdominals are pulled in tight throughout, to stabilise the spine. 4. Back hyperextensions – holding weights in hands held at shoulder level, keeping the hips, knees and feet in contact with the floor, lift the chest and arms off the floor. 5. Shuttle sprint runs – fast and slow speeds 6. Arm punching – keeping elbows bent and close to the body, swing the dumbbell forwards and back from the shoulder. Take up preferred stance – orthodox or southpaw; try changing stance between the two at various times. Each station will be performed for 30 secs, with no rest. Once all stations have been completed, move on to the next station. If, however, the circuit is a standalone activity, take a 60-second rest, then start the mini circuit again. Equipment: Skipping or speed ropes; mats; dumbbells; marker cones; sets of dumbbells (1.5–5 kg)

Cricket
Needs analysis

This game involves batting, fielding and bowling; in each of these positions there is an element of skill under pressure, be it reaction, co-ordination, agility or balance. The main energy pathway is aerobic, therefore apart from skill and technique coaching, physical fitness training needs to involve maintaining skill while using the anaerobic pathway to help the cricketer tolerate creatine depletion and lactic acid build-up.

Warm-up

The structure of the warm-up should follow the recommendations in Chapters 6 and 7. Players should be encouraged to have bat and ball and to use them to perform mobility exercises. During the stretch emphasis should be placed on hamstrings, quadriceps, back, hip flexors, pectorals and calves. Pulse-raising can be achieved by adapting exercises that take the large muscle groups through a gradual increase in their range of movement as shown in Chapter 6.

Cool-down

Some of the pulse-rising activities can be repeated post-circuit to aid removal of waste and ensure muscles are warm enough for the longer stretch. Perform stretches covering a whole body approach as described in Chapter 7, developing those areas identified in the flexibility focus.

Specific muscles used: quadriceps, hip flexors; gluteals; hamstrings; anterior tibialis; triceps; pectorals; traps

Joints used: ankles; knees; hips; spine; shoulders; elbows

Predominant energy pathway: aerobic

Flexibility focus: hip flexors; hamstrings; gastrocnemius; pectorals

Equipment required: cricket bats and balls; tennis balls; bucket; cones; spring wickets; rugby tackle bag or similar that will stand tall; mats

---

Table 16.7	Cricket circuit
Station 1	**Hit and run** Emphasis: skill; anaerobic conditioning A player hits a rugby tackle bag or similar object. Different strokes can be used and identified next to the station. Once the stroke has been made, the player then runs to a set of stumps or cones and back. Equipment: Rugby tackle bag or rolled up gym mats; cricket bat; stumps or cones
Station 2	**Chasing balls** Emphasis: anaerobic conditioning A number of tennis balls are randomly placed in a circle around a bucket. The distance from bucket to ball needs to be such to allow a challenging grid run. The players have to run to pick up a ball and place it in the bucket. When all balls have been retrieved, they then have to be returned to their starting place. The station is continuous. Equipment: Eight to ten tennis balls; bucket
Station 3	**Boundary fielding** Emphasis: anaerobic conditioning; skill Two players stand side by side (a non-participating coach can be used as the feeder if desired). The ball is fed underarm along the ground, and the player has to run and pick up the ball before it crosses the marked boundary, turn and throw back to the feeding player. If two players are used, they both run out to try and stop the ball. When the pick-up has been made they turn around and change the feeding and pick-up player. Play is continuous. Equipment: Several cricket balls
Station 4	**Between-wicket running** Emphasis: anaerobic conditioning The ends of a track are marked out by cones, with a player standing at each end with a bat in hand. On the start signal they run between the wickets, trying to catch up or overtake the other player. Counting the runs achieved in the time frame, check who wins at the end of the training session. Equipment: Marker cones; cricket bat per person; pads if possible

Table 16.7	Cricket circuit cont.
Station 5	**Catching skills** Emphasis: skill Players stand about 3 m from a flat wall. Using a tennis ball, they throw the ball against the wall and catch the rebound with the preferred hand. Repeat using the non-preferred hand, and then a mixture of both. Vary the pace at which the ball is thrown. Alternate this activity with throwing a ball at a target 30 cm from the ground and catching the rebound. Half the allotted time could be spent doing each activity. Should a catching cradle be available, use it. Equipment: Wall or catching cradle; tennis balls; cricket balls
Station 6	**Measured bowling** Emphasis: skill Using beanbags or tennis/cricket balls, aim to bounce the ball in the various targets laid out on the floor. The correct bowling action should be used and the bowler must follow through to cross a line 1.5 m from the crease. Take it in turn to bowl, or one at a time with the partner retrieving balls/bags. Change around at half time. Equipment: Bucket of balls or beanbags; wickets; marked out crease
Station 7	**Dive and catch** Emphasis: skill; anaerobic conditioning One player has a cricket ball, the other the bat, standing about 4–5 m apart. The player with the ball feeds the batsman, who hits a wide and low shot; the bowler has to dive to catch the ball. The ball has to be caught on both sides and at feet. Change around at half time. Equipment: Cricket bat; cricket balls
Station 8	**Mini-circuit** Emphasis: muscle endurance/strength (erector spinae group; transversus abdominis; obliques; rectus abdominis; gluteals; quadriceps; pectorals; triceps; rotator cuff group) Incorporating back extensions, abdominals ('the plank'), obliques, gluteals, quadriceps, pectorals and triceps and rotator cuff group (use appropriate exercises described in Chapter 11).

Cycling

Needs analysis

Cycling requires a high degree of aerobic conditioning, which can be affected by lack of local muscular endurance in the main working muscle groups (indicated right). There are various different types of cycling: road, track, mountain biking, cyclo-cross, and of course recreational cycling. The circuit has been designed with all of these in mind and will help develop muscular endurance through cycle-specific joint and muscle actions.

Warm-up

The structure of the warm-up should follow the guidelines laid out in Chapters 6 and 7. Should spinning bikes be available they could be utilised to carry out the warm-up to really make the circuit cycle-specific. Exercisers could also use their own bikes to perform this outdoors on a gradated intensity ride.

Cool-down

Back on bikes, if available, to re-warm muscles ready for final stretch. If no bikes are available, use similar exercises to the warm-up, for the purpose of building up muscle temperature in order to stretch those muscles identified in the flexibility focus.

Specific muscles used: quadriceps; gluteals; calves; hamstrings; erector spinae.

Joints used: hips; knees; ankles.

Predominant energy pathway: aerobic.

Flexibility focus: Hip flexors; hamstrings; anterior tibialis; calves; pectorals; triceps.

Equipment required: Stationary bikes; step benches; marker cones; short metal or wooden bar 30 cm long; length of cordage (90 cm); 2.5–5 kg weight; barbells with appropriate weight; mats; ankle weights.

Table 16.8	Cycling circuit
Station 1	**Stationary cycling** Emphasis: aerobic conditioning Using an upright bike (spinning bike), perform sprinting exercise. Equipment: Spinning bikes
Station 2	**The lifting phase** Emphasis: muscular strength and endurance Using ankle weights or similar, sit on a table. Leading with the knees, lift and lower the knees, under control, up to waist height, simulating the cycling action. Equipment: Table; ankle weights or similar

Table 16.8	Cycling circuit cont.
Station 3	**Squat thrusts** Emphasis: muscular strength and endurance Take up a front support position with the arms under the shoulders and a slight bend in the elbows; one leg needs to be straight and one bent, with the knee between the arms in line with the hips. Keeping the bottom high take the bent leg back and the straight leg forwards in a continuous rhythmic action.
Station 4	**The Plank** Emphasis: core stability Lie face down on the floor, keeping everything in contact with the floor and supporting the head on the back of the hands. Take a breath in and then out, pull in the belly button (umbilicus) towards the spine and hold, breathing throughout. Hold for about 10 secs then release. Repeat. Alternatively, this can be done by supporting the body on the knees and hands but making sure the back is flat. Equipment: Mats
Station 5	**Back extension** Emphasis: muscular strength and endurance Standing feet hip-width apart, take a bend at the hips and knees, keeping the knees in line with the feet and behind the toes, the bottom above the knees (thighs should be parallel with the floor). Drive up, leading with the hands and arms, and jump into the air, landing with heels on the floor back in the squat position. Repeat. Equipment: Mats; dumbbells
Station 6	**Wrist curls** Emphasis: muscular strength and endurance Hold on to a small bar with a rope tied to it. At the other end of the rope is tied a weight. Keeping the elbows locked into the sides of the body and maintaining a right angle at the elbow joint, roll the wrist and wind the rope onto the bar until it reaches the top, then reverse the action and lower the weight to the floor. Equipment: Barbell with appropriate weight; chair
Station 7	**Squat** Emphasis: muscular strength and endurance Stand with feet pedal-width apart, bending at the hips and knees and keeping the feet behind the toe line and in line with the feet. At the lowest point keep the bottom above the knees and the shoulders above the bottom. Drive through the legs and stand up. Repeat.

Table 16.8	Cycling circuit cont.
Station 8	**Hip extension** Emphasis: muscular strength and endurance Lie on the floor on the back, knees bent, and feet flat on the floor. Lift the hips off the floor, supporting the upper body on the shoulders, and fix the 'abs' tight to support the spine. Lift the hips up towards the ceiling and lower under control using a slow to moderate speed. Equipment: Mats; gym ball, if available
Station 9	**Calf raises** Emphasis: muscular strength and endurance Stand with feet hip-width apart, toes facing forwards, and keep the rest of the body in an upright position, possibly using a support to aid stability. Keeping the posture upright, lift up on to the toes while maintaining a slight bend in the knees, then return the heels to the floor and repeat.
Station 10	**Narrow support press-ups** Emphasis: muscular strength and endurance Take up the front support position with the hands close together on a bench or step under the chest, fingers facing forwards at full extension. Keep a slight bend in the elbow, and the toes on the floor. Bend the arms outwards to lower the chest to the bench. Push through the hands to achieve full extension again.
Station 11	**Shuttle runs** Emphasis: aerobic conditioning Take up a weight (dumbbells or other appropriate resistance) and run a course of obstacles to include stepping over benches, running across crash mats, etc. Equipment: Dumbbells; crash mats; gym benches
Station 12	**Single-leg step-ups** Emphasis: muscular strength and endurance Stand facing sideways on to a bench. Place one foot onto the bench then drive up through full extension with a jump, landing back on the same leg. Continue to use the same leg for a period of time then change side and leg. Equipment: Gym benches or step boxes

Football

Needs analysis

This circuit has been designed with the following elements in mind. The game has various positions that a player can be asked to play in, which include the goal. But whatever the position, the skills and conditioning required are generic. Players need muscular strength and endurance to help withstand knocks and for challenging for the ball, and explosive power for quick sprints, jumps and throws. A high level of aerobic conditioning to reduce the onset of fatigue, and both on- and off-the-ball skills, such as balance, agility, reaction and power, are required.

Warm-up

The structure of the warm-up should follow the guidelines laid out in Chapters 6 and 7. It is strongly recommended that each person should have a football or at least one between two. Mobility exercises can be performed with ball in hand (these could include throw-ins, ball juggling and hand-to-hand passing of the ball to a partner around the body), as can the pulse-raising, only this time the ball will be at the feet. These activities should encompass passing and dribbling skills at different paces, followed by small-sided games in grids. Stretching of the main muscle groups (whole body approach) should be included prior to the grid games.

Cool-down

On completion of the circuit, time permitting, a small-sided game could be included as a re-warming prior to the post-stretch. This would be followed by the stretch component as described in Chapter 7, emphasis being paid to the areas indicated in the flexibility focus.

Specific muscles used: hamstrings; adductors; hip flexors; quadriceps; gluteals.

Joints used: knees; hips; ankles; shoulders; elbows.

Predominant energy pathway: aerobic/anaerobic.

Flexibility focus: hamstrings; adductors; hip flexors; quadriceps.

Equipment required: training balls; goalmouth; gym benches; numerous marker cones; speed and agility ladder or similar; medicine balls; various weights; badminton net and posts; rubber resistance bands of various levels of resistance.

Table 16.9	Football circuit
Station 1	**Resistance kicks** Emphasis: local muscular endurance (quadriceps; hamstrings; hip flexors) Using a rubber band as the resistance, tie the two ends to an anchor point and place the foot into the loop or tie one end of the band to the anchor point and the other end to the leg around the ankle. Extend the leg, as though kicking a ball. Perform this exercise for, say, ten reps then change legs. Equipment: Rubber resistance bands
Station 2	**Shuttle maze tracking run** Emphasis: aerobic conditioning; skill Place cones 10 m apart in a zigzag fashion. The players, working in pairs, have to face each other throughout the maze run; one sprints forwards to the first cone, while the partner tracks progress running backwards, keeping within an arm's distance. Round the cone then run backwards, tracking partner running forwards. The second run is done controlling a football; this time you face the way you are going, and make sure the ball is kept in close control. Continue to alternate the maze run as indicated. Equipment: Marker cones; training football
Station 3	**Body tennis** Emphasis: skill Set up a net on two posts about chest height. Players stand either side of the net, using all parts of the body other than the arms and hands. Keep the ball from touching the ground. A maximum of three hits is allowed before the ball must pass over the net. Should the ball touch the floor then the offending player should carry out a forfeit during the changeover. Equipment: Badminton posts and net; football
Station 4	**Throw and trap** Emphasis: explosive power (abdominal region; anterior deltoids; triceps; quadriceps; hip flexors); skill Throw a medicine ball against a wall and trap the return. Replace the medicine ball with a regular ball, sprint maintaining close control and, using both feet, dribble around laid out cones, push pass against a box (fictitious player), then take the return and shoot into a goal. Equipment: Medicine ball; football; marker cones

Table 16.9	Football circuit cont.
Station 5	**Obstacle course** Emphasis: aerobic conditioning Lay out a course to include cones to form a path allowing players to side step between cones, a ladder (substitute wooden battens for the ladder for safety) so that the players can step quickly across the steps into the spaces, and tyres placed diagonally side by side for players to step into the middle of each tyre. Equipment: Marker cones; speed and agility ladder; tyres; small hurdles or equivalent 30 cm high
Station 6	**Bounders** Emphasis: explosive power (quadriceps; calves; gluteals; hamstrings) With a two-footed take off, explode into the air as high as possible, making sure to land on the opposite side of the bench. Repeat until all benches have been cleared, then sprint back to the start and repeat the bounding. Use a combination of take offs, left leg, right leg, two-footed, etc. Equipment: Gym benches or step box
Station 7	**Shuttle, dribble, sprint** Emphasis: aerobic conditioning Lay out a grid with lines or cones set at 10, 20 and 30 m from the base line. The player dribbles the ball and stops it on the 10 m line, runs backwards to the base line, sprints to the ball, picks it up and dribbles to the 20 m line. Again run backwards to the base line then repeat to the 30 m line. Then repeat the sequence in the opposite direction. Players must maintain close control of the ball during the dribbling phase and stop it dead on the line. Equipment: three marker cones; football
Station 8	**Push passing** Emphasis: local muscular endurance (adductors; hip flexors; hamstrings; abdominal region; erector spinae) Two benches or rebound boards are placed opposite each other, 15 m apart. The player stands on the centre line between the rebound boards and push passes the ball with one foot against the rebound board, trapping the return. The activity is then repeated using the other foot and the other bench. Once the pass has been performed twice with each leg, the player takes up the prone position and carries out squat thrusts for 15 secs, then repeats the push passing again, and so on. Failure to trap the ball will lead to a forfeit being carried out during the changeover. Equipment: Two wooden gym benches or rebound boards; football

Table 16.9	Football circuit cont.
Station 9	**Goalkeeping practice** Emphasis: skill; anaerobic conditioning Arrange four balls in a square or in a fan shape on the ground, 5 m apart. Place a ball in the centre of the square or level with the centre of the fan, as the home base. The player starts off by touching the ball in the centre with both hands then runs to each of the corner balls, touching them with both hands. The player has to touch the centre ball before moving to the next corner. A variety of movement between the balls can be adopted. Forwards out, backwards back, sideways out and sideways back. To aid skills, each corner could be numbered and the player go to the called number. Equipment: Five footballs
Station 10	**Goalkeeping reaction dive** Emphasis: skill The keeper faces the goal with their back to their partner, holding a ball. They bend forwards and roll the ball through their legs to the partner standing on the penalty spot or equivalent. The outfield player then shoots at the goal. The keeper has to turn and save the shot. After five shots the players change position and repeat. This activity is completed for the given time frame. Equipment: Portable goal; football

Hockey

Needs analysis

The hockey player predominately uses the aerobic energy system; however, there is a great need for the anaerobic systems (PC and lactic acid) to be trained as well. These can be trained in a non-game situation; the circuit has been designed with exercises/drills that will allow improvements in aerobic conditioning, muscular strength, power, local muscular endurance and, of course, skills such as balance, reactions and agility. Postural stability is also important and the lack of this will affect the development of muscular strength, endurance and skill.

Warm-up

The structure of the warm-up should follow the guidelines, laid out in Chapters 6 and 7. The mobility and pulse-raising activities could be carried out with sticks in hand. Pulse-raising activities should include a ball, working in pairs to pass and stop the ball on the move, left and right in front and behind the body. Prior to the more vigorous pulse-raising, such as a timed game or team relays with stick and ball, a whole body stretch should be performed as explained in Chapter 7.

Cool-down

The circuit can be finished off by playing a timed game; this can act as a re-warming activity prior to the final stretch guidelines for maintenance and developmental stretching as laid out in Chapter 7. Emphasis should be placed on the muscle groups in the flexibility focus.

Specific muscles used: calves; quadriceps; hamstrings; gluteals; erector spinae; hip flexors; deltoids; abdominals.

Joints used: Ankles; knees; hips; spine; shoulders; elbows.

Predominant energy pathway: aerobic.

Flexibility focus: erector spinae; hip flexors; hamstrings; gluteals; calves; adductors; triceps; abdominals.

Equipment required: marker cones; hockey sticks; balls; crash mats or similar; resistance harness; barbell with a selection of free weight discs; four badminton posts; four lengths of rope; rolled up gym mats or rubber tyres; various strength resistance bands; selection of dumbbells.

Table 16.10	Hockey circuit
Station 1	**Maze run** Emphasis: aerobic conditioning Run to the cones placed in a zigzag formation. At each cone, reach and touch the line marked on the floor to the side, left and right with your hockey stick. When the course has been completed, return backwards, again reaching the line left and right. Equipment: Six cones, hockey sticks and taped line
Station 2	**Abdominal circuit** Emphasis: muscular strength and endurance of the abdominal region; postural stability Perform abdominal curls, full sit-ups, oblique curls and 'the plank' while holding stick in hand. Equipment: Several mats and hockey sticks
Station 3	**Resistance running** Emphasis: aerobic conditioning Using either a crash mat or resistance harness, working in pairs carry out a shuttle sprint, or sprint on the spot if using the crash mat. Sticks must be carried. Equipment: Crash mats, resistance harness and hockey sticks
Station 4	**Bent forward rowing and back extensions** Emphasis: local muscular endurance of the back (erector spinae) Using a weight that will challenge the targeted muscle (erector spinae), dead-lift the weight and adjust the feet to shoulder-width apart for stability. Change the grip to shoulder width, keeping a slight bend in the knees and tight 'abs', then lean forwards while maintaining a long spine. Lead with the elbows and draw the weight into the lower chest. Keeping the wrist firm, return the weight to its starting position, keeping a slight bend at the elbows. Repeat. Equipment: Barbells with a selection of weight plates
Station 5	**Squat run** Emphasis: local muscular endurance of the gluteals, quadriceps and erector spinae Lay four posts out in a square with a rope tied to each post that gradually gets lower as the rope is wound around the four posts. The player has to squat under the rope from side to side, stick leading, reaching ahead to left and right alternately. Equipment: Four badminton posts; four lengths of rope and hockey sticks
Station 6	**Static hit** Emphasis: skill; explosive power of the upper back and deltoids

Table 16.10	Hockey circuit cont.
	Using a rolled up mat or rubber tyre, step in and hit the obstacle with the stick. Step back and repeat the strike. Take a pause between each strike.
	Equipment: Rolled mats or rubber tyres and hockey stick
Station 7	**Plank attack**
	Emphasis: core stability, explosive power of the leg extensors
	Performing 'the plank' exercise as on p. 130, hold the position for 10 secs then as quickly as possible get up to standing and sprint to the cone opposite; jog back and start again. The stick must be carried throughout.
	Equipment: Cones and hockey stick
Station 8	**Resistance hitting**
	Emphasis: local muscular endurance of the deltoids and upper back
	Using a rubber resistance band tied to the stick and anchored to the wall, perform continuous pushing action.
	Equipment: Rubber resistance bands and hockey sticks
Station 9	**Step lunging**
	Emphasis: local muscular endurance of the quadriceps, gluteals and back
	Standing on the centreline, side step to the next line left or right, side lunge and reach for the next line with the hockey stick. Return to the centreline and repeat to the opposite side.
	Equipment: Marker cones and hockey sticks
Station 10	**Dead-lift**
	Emphasis: muscular strength and endurance
	Selecting either a barbell or set of dumbbells with appropriate weight to challenge the targeted muscles (gluteals, quadriceps, erector spinae), stand with feet hip-width apart, toes under the bar, bending at the hips and knees, keeping the knees in line with the toes. Take hold of the bar with a shoulder-width grip. Leading with the shoulders and driving through the legs, stand up. Reverse the movement by lowering the bar to the shins, then repeat.
	Equipment: Barbells or dumbbells and appropriate weight plates
Station 11	**Whole group activity**
	Emphasis: anaerobic conditioning
	Grid sprints, gradually increasing the distance from 10 m through 20–30 m with a rest between sprints.
	Equipment: Marker cones

Netball

Needs analysis

Netball is a game of short, sharp bursts of energy with an aerobic recovery; skills such as reactions, agility and co-ordination are also needed in abundance. The following circuit has been designed to address these areas; it can be used for out of season training or indeed weekly practice training.

Warm-up

The structure of the warm-up should follow the guidelines laid out in Chapters 6 and 7. The mobility and pulse-raising could be performed with each player having a ball, or at least one between two players. The pulse-raising activities can be a gradual increase in the pace of passing and moving around the court. An exercise from Chapter 7 can be included to ensure thorough warming prior to the circuit, making sure that a whole body stretch has been performed prior to the more vigorous pulse-raising; as discussed in Chapter 7.

Cool-down

A timed game can be used to re-warm the body prior to the final stretch, guidelines of which are in Chapter 8. Make sure that development of the muscle groups identified in the flexibility focus takes place.

Specific muscles used: quadriceps; gluteals; hamstrings; calves; deltoids; triceps.

Joints used: ankles; knees; hips; spine; shoulders; elbows.

Predominant energy pathway: aerobic/anaerobic PC.

Flexibility focus: calves; hamstrings; adductors; quadriceps; deltoids; triceps.

Table 16.11	Netball Circuit
Station 1	**Reaction track** Emphasis: skill; aerobic conditioning; speed off the mark Start on a point between lines of randomly placed cones set well apart. Both players face the same direction, one behind the other. The player at the back initiates the direction and the other will try to beat them to the designated cone. After five runs, change the leading player so both get the opportunity to initiate the direction. Equipment: Ten cones
Station 2	**Loaded twisting sit-ups** Emphasis: local muscular endurance of the abdominal region Two players sit side by side on a mat, knees bent, feet flat on the floor, facing each other. Both players perform a sit-up. At the top of the movement a medicine ball is passed from one player to the other and placed on the floor. The sit-up is then performed and the medicine ball transfer is repeated. Action is continued for the set period of time. Equipment: Mats; medicine balls
Station 3	**Lunge passing** Emphasis: local muscular endurance (quadriceps, hip flexors); explosive power of the deltoids Stand on the line provided; lunge forward and chest pass a medicine ball to a partner. Ensure you alternate the leading leg when lunging to achieve muscle balance. Equipment: Medicine ball; floor markings
Station 4	**Sprint passing** Emphasis: aerobic conditioning; skill Working in pairs, each player stands behind a line of cones set 3–5 m apart. A player chest passes the ball to their partner; they then sprint to the first cone ready to receive the ball back again. Their partner chest or shoulder passes the ball back and then sprints to their next cone, and so on along the line of cones to the end. The players then work their way back to the start. Repeat. Equipment: Ten cones; netball
Station 5	**Calf raises** Emphasis: local muscular endurance of the gastrocnemius Stand on a bench or step box with the balls of the feet in contact with the top, using a wall for support. Continue to rise up and down on the toes, gradually increasing the range of movement. Equipment: Step box; wall

Table 16.11	Netball Circuit cont.
Station 6	**Power jumps** Emphasis: explosive power of the quadriceps; aerobic conditioning Three step boxes are laid out in a line. Players run out to the first box, place the leading leg on the top and drive up into the air, landing on two feet, heels down. Complete the exercise until all boxes have been jumped, jog back and start again. Equipment: Three step boxes
Station 7	**Power pass** Emphasis: local muscular endurance of the abdominal region; explosive power of the triceps and deltoids; skill Lie on the back, knees bent, feet flat on the floor, holding a medicine ball. Perform a sit-up and chest pass the ball to a partner seated on the floor opposite, who does the same to return the ball. Repeat.
Station 8	**Power jumps** Emphasis: aerobic conditioning plus explosive power of the quadriceps Using a crash mat, perform star jumps. Equipment: Crash mats

Rowing

Needs analysis

There is no substitute for rowing other than getting on the water. However, this is not always possible due to incorrect tideway conditions, weather or no boat available. To meet these unforeseen or planned periods off the water, the following activities can be performed indoors to meet the needs of the rower. It's all well and good just getting on an indoor rowing machine and hammering out the kilometres, but should there not be enough for all to use, the following exercises can be performed as a circuit to aid performance on the water. Apart from aerobic conditioning, there is a great requirement for local muscular endurance in the muscle groups listed below. Strength plays a massive part in this sport and should also be catered for. Stabilising the core muscles will aid the development of both strength and endurance, and help the rower improve their power to drive a boat forwards while reducing fatigue.

Warm-up

The structure of the warm-up should follow the guidelines laid down in Chapters 6 and 7. Though mobility of all joints to be used should be encouraged, pulse-raising using exercises described in Chapter 6 can be enhanced by incorporating partner lifting, carrying or resistance-pulling activities. A whole body stretch is recommended.

Cool-down

Some form of whole body re-warming should be carried out to ensure muscles are warm enough for the post-workout stretch. This can be achieved by repeating some of the exercises used in the pulse-raising using predominantly large muscle group actions. This can then be followed by a stretch to either maintain range of movement or develop and improve as discussed in Chapter 7.

Specific muscles used: quadriceps; gluteals; hamstrings; latissimus dorsi; trapezius; biceps; wrist flexors and extensors.

Joints used: knees; hips; shoulders; elbows.

Predominant energy pathway: aerobic

Flexibility focus: hamstrings; quadriceps; hip flexors; calves; pectoralis; triceps.

Equipment required: Concept 2 or similar; numerous gym benches or step benches; gym mats; various rubber resistance bands; 10 m of rope; weighted sliding mat; short metal or wooden bar 30 cm long; length of cordage (90 cm); 2.5–5 kg weight; barbells with appropriate weight.

Table 16.12	Rowing Circuit
Station 1	**Rowing** Emphasis: anaerobic/aerobic conditioning, dependent on duration and intensity Using a rowing ergometer, maintain a set stroke rate, which, dependent on the time on the exercise station, must challenge the body (suggest in excess of 30 SPM). Equipment: Concept 2 rowing machine or similar
Station 2	**Bench bounding** Emphasis: muscle strength/power (gastrocnemius; quadriceps; gluteals) Facing several lines of benches with a substantial gap between them, using a two-footed take-off, leap upwards and over each bench in turn without rest. Once the course has been completed, jog back to the start and repeat. Equipment: five gym benches or step boxes
Station 3	**Seated row** Emphasis: postural endurance; muscle endurance (biceps; trapezius; latissimus dorsi; posterior deltoid; rhomboids) Using rubber bands or equivalent, sit on a mat with legs out straight, back upright, and maintain good stability of the spine. Wrap the band around the feet, taking hold of each end, and perform the rowing action at a slow to moderate speed. Equipment: Rubber resistance bands; gym mats

Table 16.12	Rowing Circuit cont.
Station 4	**Drive slide** Emphasis: muscle strength/endurance (quadriceps); postural endurance Sit on a mat that will slide across the floor or equivalent material. Sit with legs bent and feet flat on the floor. Push and straighten the legs, maintaining alignment of hips, knees and feet, driving the mat and body across the floor. When the end of the course has been reached, turn around and push yourself back. Repeat. If more than one person is on this station it could be conducted as a race against each other. Equipment: Sliding mat or material
Station 5	**Resistance pulling** Emphasis: muscle endurance (biceps; trapezius; latissimus dorsi; posterior deltoid; rhomboids) Working on your own or with a partner, take up a sitting position opposite a weighted mat on the other side of the hall. A rope is attached to the mat on either side. The seated exerciser takes hold of the rope and pulls the mat across the hall using only the arms and back. There should be no excessive rotational movement of the spine during this action. Once the mat has reached the puller, they then jog to the other side and repeat the action. If working in pairs there will be a recovery phase, while the other partner pulls. Equipment: Long length of rope; weighted sliding mat
Station 6	**Power clean or High pull** Emphasis: muscle strength/endurance (gastrocnemius; quadriceps; hamstrings; gluteals; erector spinae; biceps; trapezius; deltoid) Use a barbell, with a weight that is appropriate to challenge the exerciser. Perform 'the clean' continuously for a given number of reps and sets within the given time frame for each station. 'The clean' must be performed with correct technique. Should this not be possible, the high pull can be used, which only takes the weight to shoulder height with a hip-width grip and elbows high. Equipment: Barbells with a selection of weight plates
Station 7	**Weight winding** Emphasis: muscle endurance (wrist flexors/extensors) Use a bar approximately 18 in long with a length of rope tied to the middle of it and a weight on the other end. Several bars can be provided with different weight loads. Stand with feet hip-width apart to give stability, take hold of the bar at each end, and curl the wrists to wind the weight up. When the weight has reached the top, reverse the action under control. The exercise can be performed in several ways – arms outstretched, elbows locked by the side or a combination of both. Equipment: Short metal/wooden bar; length of cordage; 2.5–5 kg plates

Table 16.12	Rowing Circuit cont.
Station 8	**Bent over rowing** Emphasis: muscle endurance/strength (trapezius; rhomboids; posterior deltoid; latissimus dorsi; biceps; brachialis) Using a barbell, perform the following exercise. Stand with feet hip-width apart, take a shoulder-width grip of the bar and, maintaining alignment of hips, knees and ankles, dead-lift the bar. Take a slight lean forwards, being sure to maintain spine stability. Push the weight forwards and then leading with the elbows pull the bar into the abdominal region, keeping the wrists firm throughout. Repeat for the desired number of repetitions to achieve a training effect. Equipment: Barbell bars with a selection of weight plates
Station 9	**Pull-ups** Emphasis: muscle strength/endurance (latissimus dorsi; biceps; brachialis) This exercise can only be performed if a suitable 'chinning' bar is available. Take an overhand grip of the bar/beam pull and lift the body up until the chin has passed the bar/beam. Lower fully without touching the floor under control. Should a bar/beam not be available, the exercise can be performed using a rubber band wrapped around an anchor point. Lie on the floor face down, taking the ends of the band in each hand. Starting with a wide arm and leading with the elbows, draw the arms down and into the side (adduction), similar to the 'lats pull down' exercise. Equipment: Chinning bar or equivalent; rubber resistance bands
Station 10	**Core stability** Emphasis: muscle endurance of above muscle groups Abdominal and erector spinae exercises can be performed as a whole group at the end of the above exercises. The following stations are suggested and one or two may be selected: 'the plank' (for transverses), abdominal curls (for rectus abdominis) and oblique curls (for obliques). Back hyperextensions can be used for the back. There may be a need to include exercises that balance muscle groups used in the circuit, such as pecs (bench flyes), triceps (dips or push downs). Equipment: Mats; gym balls if available; dumbbells; step benches; rubber resistance bands

Rugby

Needs analysis

The game of rugby requires its players to give maximum output for the whole duration of the game; therefore a high level of aerobic conditioning is required, whatever position is played. This will help reduce the build-up of lactic acid in the muscles. Training specific muscles as indicated for improvements in strength and endurance will help a player develop power (strength) for scrummaging, rucking and mauls. Endurance training or a combination of both will help players to continue to exert force over time. The circuit has been designed to work the anaerobic pathways, namely the PC and lactic acid systems.

Warm-up

The structure of the warm-up should follow the guidelines laid out in Chapters 6 and 7. It is strongly recommended that each person should have a ball, or at least one between two. Mobility exercises can be performed with ball in hand; these could include hand-to-hand passing of the ball to a partner, incorporating around the body, through the legs and overhead passing; putting the ball to the ground and picking up should help mobilise the lower body and act as a pulse-raising exercise. Further pulse-raising can be carried out by including passing while on the move or partner pulling/pushing type movements. For further exercises see Chapters 6 and 7. A whole body stretch should be included before the more intense/vigorous activities commence.

Cool-down

At the end of the circuit a timed game of touch rugby can be used as the re-warming in preparation for the post-stretch. Ensure a whole body stretch is performed as recommended in Chapter 13, with emphasis on developing the range of movement of those muscles and joints identified in the flexibility focus.

Specific muscles used: gluteals; quadriceps; hamstrings; calves; abductors; adductors; anterior tibialis; erector spinae; trapezius; pectorals; deltoids.

Joints used: ankles; knees; hips; spine; shoulders; elbows.

Predominant energy pathway: aerobic/anaerobic – power.

Flexibility focus: hamstrings; hip flexors; calves; gluteals; quadriceps; anterior tibialis; pectoralis; trapezius.

Equipment required: training balls; tackle bags or equivalent; mats; suspended balls.

Table 16.13	Rugby Circuit
Station 1	**The side step** Emphasis: aerobic/muscle endurance; skill Tackle bags or cones are laid out in a line, placed so that the player cannot run around them. The player starts about 5 m from the obstacles, runs, picks up a ball from the floor halfway, then side steps the tackle bags to the other end of the course where the ball is placed on the floor. Repeat the exercise in the opposite direction, only this time throw dummy passes during the side steps. Equipment: Rugby tackle bags or equivalent; training balls
Station 2	**The scrummage** Emphasis: muscular strength and endurance; gluteals; quadriceps Both players stand back to back in a designated zone. One of the players gives the signal and they hop to a line 5 m away, turn and hop back using the other leg. They then take up a scrummage position against each other, making sure they keep a flat, strong, back position and push against each other across a line 2 m away. Once the line has been crossed, it's back to the start zone and the whole thing is repeated. For variety, instead of pushing, the scrummage could be wheeled ninety degrees.
Station 3	**The tackle** Emphasis: skill; muscular strength and endurance Players start this activity on their knees and practise tackling each other from the side, back and front. This activity can be progressed to standing, with the tackler taking up a crouched position through walking to a jog. When the tackle is made at speed, use tackle bags. The other important aspect of this practice is getting up from the tackle, ready for the next. Equipment: Gym mats; tackle bag
Station 4	**The maul** Emphasis: muscular strength and endurance One player has the ball in a standing position, the main objective to resist being turned or pushed back. The other player has to lift and turn the player using a bear hug, then push the player and the ball across a line. Once across the line they then have to try and rip the ball from the grasp of their partner. This is all done within a time frame; regardless of outcome, when time is up players change positions. Equipment: Training balls; marker cones
Station 5	**Defensive pick-up** Emphasis: explosive leg power A ball is fed forwards with pace. After the feed is made one of the players has to run drop on the ball, back towards their goal line. Pick up ball and run back to the start. Roles are then changed. Repeat. Equipment: Training balls; marker cones

Table 16.13	Rugby Circuit cont.

Station 6	**The line out** Emphasis: explosive leg power A line of balls are, if possible, suspended from above at varying heights from 3 m up to 5 m. Players stand in normal line out formation ready to receive the ball. One player jumps to touch the ball with both hands while the other player(s) lift and assist the catch. Each ball has to be touched in turn. Repeat, changing the jumping player. Equipment: Training balls; means of suspending balls from above
Station 7	**Partner resistance circuit** Emphasis: muscular strength and endurance A variety of pulling and pushing activities are to be performed one after the other. Each time around the circuit, where necessary, partners will take it in turns to lead. Pulling exercises: • holding onto each other's wrists – a single-arm pull to cross a line • interlock elbows – pull partner across a line • double arm hold of wrists – pull partner across a line. Resistance running: Wrap a piece of rope harness around the waist of the running partner, who has to shuttle run over a given distance in excess of 10 m. The other partner holding the rope resists the runner. Either a pulled tyre can substitute the harness, or a weighted mat, or even a small parachute. Pushing exercises: • use a large tackle bag or rolled up mat held between the players, push each other to cross a line • hopping on one leg, hand on partner's head, hop and push partner across line • hopping with arms folded, hop and push partner across line. Equipment: Vehicle tyre; drag parachute; harness; tackle bag
Station 8	**Press-up and get-up** Emphasis: muscular strength and endurance A row of balls are placed on the ground 1 m apart. One player takes up the front support position over the first ball. The partner stands about 3 m away to receive a pass. Perform five press-ups, quickly, stand up with the ball, pass to partner and move on to the next ball. Repeat the press-ups, during which each ball passed is replaced on its spot. Once all balls have been passed, partners change places. Speed of getting up and accuracy of the pass are as important as good technique press-ups. Equipment: Minimum of five training balls

Skiing

Needs analysis

There are different disciplines within skiing: downhill, cross-country and slalom. The following circuit is designed more for the recreational skier, although they can be adapted for the serious performer. The skier requires a high level of muscular strength and endurance conditioning; this will help them maintain muscular contractions for longer, reducing the build-up of lactic acid, while still being able to exert force. The need for balance and co-ordination while on skis has also been catered for.

Warm-up

The structure of the warm-up should follow the guidelines laid out in Chapters 6 and 7. Ski poles, if available, can be used during the mobility component to add realism. The pulse-raising activities should closely resemble ski movements using large (leg) muscles predominately; adopt a whole body approach when stretching.

Cool-down

To ensure all muscle groups have enough warmth in them to safely and effectively stretch, carry out similar exercises as used in the warm-up. The post-stretch should follow the guidelines laid down in Chapter 7, paying particular attention to those muscle groups in the flexibility focus.

Specific muscles used: quadriceps; gluteals; abdominal region; erector spinae; pectorals; latissimus dorsi; trapezius; deltoids.

Joints used: knees; ankles; hips; spine; shoulders.

Predominant energy pathway: aerobic/anaerobic (lactic acid).

Flexibility focus: hamstrings; adductors; calves; abductors; gluteals; hip flexors; deltoids.

Equipment required: gym mats; ski poles; various wooden gym benches or equivalent; rubber resistance bands of various resistance; dumbbells; stairway.

Table 16.14	Skiing Circuit
Station 1	**Twist jumps** Emphasis: muscular strength and endurance; quadriceps; gluteals Keeping feet fixed together, jump upwards and twist in mid-air to the right. On landing make sure that both feet are still together with heels on the floor. Bend at the knees and touch the floor with the right hand, just behind the outside of the heel. Repeat the exercise with the jump twist to the left. Make the jumps to the right and left continuous.
Station 2	**Falling down and standing up** Emphasis: muscular strength and endurance Standing between two mats, keeping the feet together, fall sideways and land on the mat. Using poles or similar for support, regain the standing position, making sure the feet stay together. Repeat the exercise on the other side. Make the falls to the left and right continuous. Equipment: Gym mats or crash mats; ski poles or similar
Station 3	**Side stepping** Emphasis: muscular strength and endurance; abductors and adductors; skill Tie a rubber resistance band around the ankles (allow some give). Stand with feet together and the right or left shoulder facing the course. Negotiate the obstacles by only taking side steps. The course should comprise of benches to step across and up onto. A stairway can be used provided it's not in use by others. At the end of the course, the skiers should walk back to the start taking large steps, then repeat the course. Equipment: Rubber resistance bands; gym benches; step boxes and stairway
Station 4	**Pole work** Emphasis: muscular strength and endurance – upper body Hold on to two rubber resistance bands anchored at one end behind or in front of the skier. Stand and simulate the pushing action, either single-arm, both arms together or a combination of both. Skiers must feel the resistance. The resistance bands can be substituted by dumbbells. Equipment: Selection of rubber resistance bands; sets of dumbbells 1.5–5 kg; ski poles or similar
Station 5	**Side leg swings and tuck position hold** Emphasis: muscular strength and endurance – lower body Stand with feet hip-width apart, keeping the legs straight and feet facing forwards. Swing from the hips, leading with the outstep and taking the right leg out to the side then back to hip width. Repeat action using the left leg. Once five swings to either side have been completed, stand with feet and knees together, take up the tuck position and pulse, up and down either side.

Table 16.14	Skiing Circuit cont.
	Keep the upper arms tucked into the side, elbows bent as if holding poles, 'abs' tight and a strong back. Perform fifteen reps in that position then go back to the previous exercise and repeat. To add intensity during the schussing, on reps five and twelve jump to full body extension. Be sure to land with knees bent and heels down.
Station 6	**Bench jumps** Emphasis: explosive power of legs; skill Keeping the body upright and over the bench, perform double-footed jumps diagonally over the bench. Continue along the entire length of the bench. At the end turn around and walk back to the start and repeat. Equipment: Wooden gym bench or row of step boxes
Station 7	**Balance squat** Emphasis: skill; muscular strength and endurance – legs Using an overturned wooden bench, the lines marked on a sports hall floor or similar, walk along the line toe to heel. With every step made perform a squat and maintain balance. At the end of the bench turn around and do the same back along the bench. Repeat. Equipment: Wooden gym bench or 10 cm square piece of timber
Station 8	**Mini-circuit** Emphasis: muscular strength and endurance – lower body Lay the following exercises out in a circle. Individuals perform the exercises for a given time frame (15–30 secs) then move on to the next. Crouch jumping – backwards and forwards jumping over two lines or ski poles set 0.5–1 m apart. Skier starts off in between the poles. Snow plough jumps – stand in-between two lines or ski poles with feet either together or hip-width apart. Jump to a snow plough position outside of the lines, bottom down. Twist jumps – jump with both legs together and twist the upper body in the opposite direction to the legs. Edging – starting in the upright position, move to rest on the left side of the feet while maintaining balance and keeping the upper body upright. Repeat to the other side. Equipment: Ski poles

Swimming – Land Conditioning

Needs analysis

Swimming requires the performer to develop a high level of aerobic conditioning and local muscular endurance in the specific muscle groups mentioned below, in order to exert force against a resistance (water) for a continued period of time while delaying the onset of fatigue (lactic acid). Should sprinting be required then the PC anaerobic pathway needs to be trained for the development of power and strength. The following circuit can form part of an overall training programme where land training should feature. It can be performed prior to or following a swim session or as an additional training day.

Warm-up

The structure of the warm-up should follow the guidelines laid out in Chapters 6 and 7. Thorough mobility of the joints identified above is necessary to reduce risk of injury. If the circuit is being set up around a pool deck, then a swim over a certain distance using a variety of strokes can be used to induce the necessary warming effect. A whole body stretch as described in Chapter 7 should be included prior to the more vigorous pulse-raising activities.

Cool-down

Again, the pool can be used to re-warm the body prior to the final stretch, or the exercises described in Chapters 6 and 7 can be used, but this time remember to gradually taper off the range of movement (intensity). This should be followed by improving the range of movement (developmental stretching) of necessary muscle groups as indicated in the flexibility focus.

Specific muscles used: gluteals; hamstrings; biceps; latissimus dorsi; pectorals; deltoids.

Joints used: shoulders; thoracic spine; hips; ankles; elbows.

Predominant energy pathway: aerobic/anaerobic – lactic acid/PC.

Flexibility focus: pectorals; latissimus dorsi; trapezius; triceps; erector spinae; hip flexors.

Equipment required: dumbbells of various weights; step benches; rubber resistance bands of various intensity grades; sturdy table or similar; high pulley resistance machine if available; pull-ups bar if available.

Table 16.15	Swimming – Land Conditioning Circuit
Station 1	**Leg kicks** Emphasis: muscular endurance; gluteals; hamstrings Lie face down on top of a bench or step box, supported from the waist upwards. Kick legs from the hips at various tempos – either dolphin or flutter. Ankle weights can be added to increase the intensity (if doing this, be sure to maintain a slight bend at the knee joint). Equipment: Gym benches or step boxes; ankle weights
Station 2	**Straight-arm pull** Emphasis: muscular strength and endurance; latissimus dorsi; core stability Use a resistance band or rope and pulley anchored to the wall, or similar. Stand with feet shoulder-width apart and knees slightly bent, lean forwards ensuring good spine stability by pulling in the abdominals, or lie on a bench or step box which will allow a good range of movement under the body. Start with the arms outstretched above the head, take hold of each end of the resistance and pull using the appropriate stroke pattern and recovery. Throughout the range of movement keep a bend in the elbow joints so as to reduce the risk of injury. Equipment: Resistance rubber bands; gym benches or step boxes
Station 3	**Up and out** Emphasis: muscular strength and endurance – triceps Using a table or fixed support of similar height, kneel down and place both hands shoulder-width apart with elbows higher than wrists on top of the support. Keeping the chest close to the bench, press on the support and raise the body on to full extension of the arms (with a slight bend in the elbow joints). Lower under control to the start position. Repeat. Equipment: Table or similar supporting structure
Station 4	**Squat jumps** Emphasis: explosive power; gluteals; quadriceps; gastrocnemius Standing with feet hip-width apart, take a bend at the hips and knees, keeping the knees in line with the feet and behind the toes, bottom above knees (thighs should be parallel with the floor). Drive up, leading with the hands and arms and jump into the air, landing with heels on the floor back in the squat position. Repeat.
Station 5	**Back extension** Emphasis: muscular strength and endurance – erector spinae Lie face down, keeping hips, knees and feet in contact with the ground. Lift the chest and arms up off the floor and lower. This exercise is to be performed under control using slow to moderate speed. The arms can be placed in various positions to increase the intensity, or add dumbbells. Equipment: Mats; dumbbells 1.5–3 kg

Table 16.15	Swimming – Land Conditioning Circuit cont.
Station 6	**Triceps extension** Emphasis: muscular strength and endurance – triceps Use a resistance band or dumbbells, standing or seated. Place the dumbbell above the head, holding with either one or two hands; if using a resistance band, hold with one hand above the head, the other hand is held behind the back, holding onto the band as an anchor point. Starting with a bent arm, elbow pointing to the roof, extend the arm to full extension keeping a slight bend at the elbow. Then lower under control to the start position. Equipment: Resistance rubber bands or dumbbells; chairs
Station 7	**Bench flyes** Emphasis: muscular strength and endurance – pectorals Lie on the back on a bench or a gym ball with feet flat on the floor using either resistance bands or dumbbells. Start with the arms straight above the chest, holding on to the resistance. Leading with the elbows, keeping the elbow joints slightly bent, take the resistance out and away to the side, ensuring a right angle between the torso and the upper arms. Continue this outward action until the hands are out of the peripheral vision, then bring the hands and resistance back to the start position, leading with the knuckles. Repeat. Equipment: Rubber resistance bands or dumbbells of appropriate weight; step box; gym bench or gym ball
Station 8	**Pull-ups** Emphasis: muscular strength and endurance; latissimus dorsi; biceps Use a fixed bar/beam set at either seated or standing height. Take an overhand shoulder-width grip of the beam at full extension of the arm. Keeping a rigid body position, bend at the elbows and lift the chin to the bar. Slowly lower under control, then repeat. Equipment: Chinning bar; gymnasium beam; assisted chins machine or lats pull down machine, if available
Station 9	**Pull-downs** Emphasis: muscular strength and endurance; latissimus dorsi Use a resistance band anchored to a point above the head or free weights bars. Take a wide grip, holding onto either end of the band. Leading with the elbows, pull the elbows down and backwards, returning to the start position under control. Repeat. Equipment: Rubber resistance band; high pulley machine, if available
Station 10	**Abdominal exercises** Emphasis: muscular strength and endurance; abdominals and core stability · Perform a mixture of different abdominal exercises such as:

Table 16.15	Swimming – Land Conditioning Circuit cont.
	'The plank' – lie face down on the floor, keeping everything in contact with the floor and supporting the head on the back of the hands. Take a breath in and then out, pull in the belly button (umbilicus) towards the spine and hold, breathing throughout. Hold for about 10 secs, then release. Repeat. Alternatively, this can be done supporting the body on the knees and hands but making sure the back is flat. Abdominal curl – lie on the back (supine) with knees bent and feet flat on the floor. Keeping the 'abs' held tight and maintaining a gap between the chin and the chest, lift the shoulders off the floor. The arms can either be placed on the thighs, across the chest or level with the temples. Lower the body back towards the floor until the shoulders touch, and then repeat. During this exercise keep the belly button (umbilicus) pulled in tight. Oblique curl – lie on the back (supine) with knees bent and feet flat on the floor. Keeping the 'abs' held tight and maintaining a gap between the chin and the chest, lift the shoulders off the floor and, keeping one elbow in contact with the floor, twist the upper body from the waist. Return to the floor and repeat on the other side. Equipment: Mats; gym ball
Station 11	**Burpee** Emphasis: muscular strength and endurance; core stability; gluteals; hip flexors Stand in an upright position, with feet hip-width apart facing forwards. Bend the hips and knees into the squat position, simultaneously placing the hands on the floor under the shoulders. Keeping the bottom high, shoot both legs backwards, keeping the heels off the floor. Leading with the knees, keeping them in line with the hips, bring the knees back in-between the arms back into the squat position. Leading with the shoulders and driving through the legs, stand up. Repeat.
Station 12	**Squat thrusts** Emphasis: muscular strength and endurance Take up a front support position with the arms under the shoulders and a slight bend in the elbows. One leg needs to be straight and one bent with the knee between the arms in line with the hips. Keeping the bottom high, take the bent leg back and the straight leg forwards in a continuous rhythmic action.
Station 13	**Step-ups** Emphasis: muscular strength and endurance Stand facing a bench or step set at a height of 50–60 cm or appropriate to fitness level. Step on to the bench with the leading leg, making sure to use a heel-through-toe action; the whole of the foot should be on the bench. Step up with the trailing leg, aiming to achieve full extension through the legs and body. Step off, landing on the floor with a toe–heel action one foot at a time, then repeat. Try to change the leading leg by taking the last leg off the box as the first up. To increase the intensity, use dumbbells. Equipment: Step box or gym bench; dumbbells

Table 16.15	Swimming – Land Conditioning Circuit cont.
Station 14	**Reverse flyes** Emphasis: muscular strength and endurance; trapezius Kneel on a mat on one leg, leaning forwards, supporting the upper body on the thigh of the kneeling leg. Keep the arms straight with a slight bend in the elbow. Using dumbbells as the resistance, draw the shoulder blades together with no movement of the arms. This exercise can also be performed sitting in a chair. Equipment: Sets of dumbbells of various weights; mats

Volleyball

Needs analysis

The game requires its players to serve, dig and volley, jump and dive to attack opponents, and defend their half of the court. Players need to use such skills as balance, coordination and have good reactions. This circuit is based around these skills and the need to train the major muscles to produce explosive power for jumping and serving, and improve the muscular strength and endurance of the whole body.

Warm-up

The structure of the warm-up should follow the guidelines laid out in Chapters 6 and 7. Mobility exercises can be performed with or without a ball, but ideally the pulse-raising component should be with a ball. This can be done in groups of two or three, using volleying and digging techniques, ensuring the large leg muscles are used through gradual increased range of movement. Stretching of all muscle groups should be carried out prior to the more vigorous warming activities. These could take the form of net practice (dig, volley and smash) or a timed game.

Cool-down

A timed game can be used to re-warm the body, or alternatively exercises described in Chapter 7 are useful in preparing the relevant muscles for final stretching. Place the emphasis on those in the flexibility focus.

Specific muscles used: gluteals; hamstrings; calves; abdominals; trapezius; deltoids; triceps; wrist flexors/extensors.

Joints used: ankles; knees; hips; shoulders; elbows.

Predominant energy pathway: anaerobic (PC/lactic acid systems)/aerobic.

Flexibility focus: calves; hamstrings; adductors; abductors; anterior tibialis; hip flexors; pectorals.

Equipment required: equivalent of two courts; mats; dumbbells and barbells with appropriate weight for exercise; training balls; rubber resistance bands of varying resistance.

Table 16.16	Volleyball circuit
Station 1	**Shuttle running** Emphasis: aerobic conditioning Using the whole court, sprint to the 6 m line, jog/walk back, sprint to the halfway line, jog/walk back, sprint to the 12 m line, jog/walk back, and finally sprint to the 18 m line, jog/walk back. Then repeat the activity, only this time only half the court is used. Players face forwards the whole time, jogging/walking backwards to the start. Equipment: Marker cones; 18 m track if no court available
Station 2	**The smash** Emphasis: explosive power (legs; pectorals; triceps); skill Standing back to the wall, hold on to the tied rubber band, which is anchored to the wall at about shoulder height. The non-striking arm should reach up towards the ball; the striking arm is bent at the elbow, with the hand holding the rubber band past the ear, with the elbow pointing forwards. The back is slightly arched so that it can be used for extra power to smash the ball. Extend the bent arm, holding the band as if performing a smash. Repeat for ten repetitions, rest then repeat. Equipment: Rubber resistance bands of varying resistance
Station 3	**The diving dig** Emphasis: skill under pressure One player feeds the ball to a point marked on the floor/mat. The receiving player tries to retrieve the ball before it touches the floor by diving and digging the ball into the air. They then have to regain the starting position before the next ball is sent in. Repeat the drill for a given time frame then change around. Equipment: Training balls; mats
Station 4	**The single block** Emphasis: explosive power (gluteals; quadriceps; calves) Place a piece of string, net height along the wall. Players stand facing the wall; they take a two-footed take-off and reach up over the net to push off the wall. This action should be continuous for 10 secs with a 15-second rest before the drill is repeated. Equipment: Posts, nets and wall
Station 5	**The double block** Emphasis: anaerobic conditioning; skill

Table 16.16	Volleyball circuit cont.
	Similar to the above, only played on court. Players stand in the centre of the court at the net. When the attack side has been called, both players side step and set the block. Once the block is on, the players return to the centre net again and repeat the action. Alternate sides should be used when setting the block. This activity is carried out continuously within the given time frame. Equipment: Court; posts; net
Station 6	**Volley and dig tennis** Emphasis: skill; aerobic conditioning Players stand either side of a net set at the correct height. The first player throws the ball in the air, and then volleys the return over the net. The receiving player digs the return into the air and follows this up with a volley over the net. Continue until play breaks down, then start again and try and beat the previous score. To make the drill more demanding, once the ball has left the volleying player's hand, they have to retreat to the backcourt line, and get back in place to take the return pass. Equipment: Posts; net; training balls
Station 7	**Mini-circuit** The following exercises can be laid out to form a circuit: **Wrist curls** Emphasis: muscular strength and endurance of the wrist flexors Use a barbell. Take a seated position and hold a barbell just in front of the knees with the forearms resting on the thighs. The wrists are curled towards the body then away towards the floor. Equipment: Barbell and selection of weight plates; chairs **Triceps extension** Emphasis: muscular strength and endurance of the triceps Hold a barbell overhead with arms straight, wrists firm and a slight bend in the elbows. Bend at the elbows, lowering the bar down behind the head, while maintaining a fixed upper arm position. Then straighten the arm to full extension. This action should be performed using controlled movement. Equipment: Barbell and a selection of weight plates

Table 16.16	Volleyball circuit cont.

The dead-lift
Emphasis: muscular strength and endurance of the gluteals; quadriceps; erector spinae

Use a barbell, with a weight similar to your own body weight. Stand with feet hip-width apart, toes facing forwards under the bar. Bend at the hips and the knees, keeping the knees behind the toes and in line with the feet. The bottom must stay above the hips and below the shoulders. Take an overhand shoulder-width grip of the bar. To lift the bar from the floor, lead with the shoulders and drive through the legs until the legs are at full extension, with a slight bend at the knees. Lower the bar to shin level then repeat the lift.

Equipment: Barbells and a selection of weight plates

Calf raises
Emphasis: muscular strength and endurance of the gastrocnemius and soleus

Using either a set of dumbbells held in the hand or a barbell resting on the shoulders, rise up onto the toes, and then return to the floor. To increase the range of movement, place a block down to rest the front of the feet on or use a step box.

Equipment: A selection of dumbbells; step box

Station 8

Serving
Emphasis: skill; muscular endurance; deltoids; triceps

Stand a minimum of 9 m away from a wall, with the top of the net marked on it. The players serve the ball to clear the net using a variety of serving styles. Should a court be available, this would best be done to ensure the service does not go out of court. A digging practice could be included to return service.

Equipment: Training balls; wall or playing court

Station 9

Net approach
Emphasis: explosive power of the legs; muscular endurance of the abdominal region; skill

Players start by lying on their back, knees bent and feet flat on the floor. They perform sit-ups for a given number of repetitions. When completed, they stand up and make an approach to the net and jump as high as they can, as if they were either smashing or blocking. They then return to the mat, only this time lying on their front and performing back extensions. Again, once the prescribed number of repetitions has been completed, stand up and do a smash or block approach and try to beat the previous height gained. Continue the exercise, alternating the mat exercises.

Equipment: Mats; posts and net

Walking

Needs analysis

This is an indoor circuit for a group of recreational walkers who, maybe due to inclement weather, are unable to get outside to walk. The exercises are aimed at improving muscular strength and endurance of the postural muscles and general aerobic conditioning, while allowing repetition of activities to help develop correct walking skills at different speeds and techniques.

Warm-up

The structure of the warm-up should follow the guidelines laid out in Chapters 6 and 7. Mobility and pulse-raising can be combined, and most if not all should be done on the move as if out on a walk. Stretching can be incorporated in the pulse-raising prior to the more vigorous walking activities.

Cool-down

Prior to the final stretching activities, further pulse-raising can be performed to re-warm the body. A series of different length grids can be used for different speeds of walking, gradually increasing and decreasing the pace, ending up with a series of stretches to maintain range of movement and increase as necessary. Chapter 13 has clear guidelines for these activities.

Specific muscles used: tibialis anterior; calves; hamstrings; hip flexors; quadriceps; pectorals; trapezius; deltoids.

Joints used: ankles; knees; hips; shoulders.

Predominant energy pathway: aerobic.

Flexibility focus: tibialis anterior; calves; hamstrings; hip flexors; quadriceps; pectorals; trapezius; deltoids.

Equipment required: step benches; mats; beanbags or dumbbells; gym benches; marking cones.

Table 16.17	Walking circuit
Station 1	**Stepping obstacle** Emphasis: aerobic; skill Place a number of benches in line with enough space between to step into. Try where possible to have the benches at varying heights, to allow safe stepping. The walker starts at one end and walks over each bench, leading with the knee and maintaining a heel-through-toe action. At the end of the course the walker turns around and speed walks down the outside back to the start. Equipment: Adjustable step boxes
Station 2	**Carry shuttle relays** Emphasis: aerobic Beanbags, balls or small exercise mats are placed at one end of a hall/course. The walkers pick up an object and firstly walk at a pace that is faster than normal, to the other end of the

Table 16.17	**Walking circuit cont.**
	course, where they place their object in a box/area. They then walk back to the start at a faster pace, while maintaining correct walking technique. Other drills can be included in this shuttle, like walking to one end on toes or walking on heels only, even walking backwards to give certain muscle groups a rest.
	Equipment: To carry as indicated in the text
Station 3	**Back extension exercise**
	Emphasis: muscular strength and endurance; core stability
	Lying face down flat on the floor, hands can either be placed on the bottom, under the chin or out in front (dependent on fitness level). Keeping the hips, knees and feet in contact with the floor, lift the chest and arms 6–12 inches off the floor, lower under control, then repeat.
	Equipment: Gym mats; dumbbells 1.5–3 kg
Station 4	**Step this way**
	Emphasis: aerobic
	Arrange several step boxes at different heights in a fan shape. The walkers visit each bench and perform four complete step-ups at each bench, then move onto the next one. To increase the intensity of this exercise, instead of stepping onto the box with a hip-width step, use a wide 'V' step.
	Equipment: Equal number of adjustable steps to participants
Station 5	**Abdominal exercise**
	Emphasis: muscular strength and endurance; core stability
	Any abdominal exercises can be performed here to work rectus abdominis, obliques and transversus. Selection will depend on fitness level.
	Equipment: Gym mats; weights plates 5–10 kg
Station 6	**Three-legged walk**
	Emphasis: aerobic; skill
	With legs tied together around the ankles, walk the course indicated, trying to maintain a steady pace throughout. An ideal drill to help maintain a forward and back piston arm action.
	Equipment: Material for ties

Table 16.17	Walking circuit cont.
Station 7	**Press-ups** Emphasis: muscular strength and endurance; core stability; triceps; pectorals Dependent on fitness level, the press-up can be performed in any appropriate position: full, three-quarter or box position. Equipment: Gym mats

REFERENCES

ACSM (2000) 6th Edition. *ACSM's Guidelines for Exercise Testing and Prescription. USA:* Lippincott, Williams and Wilkins.

ACSM (2005) 7th Edition. *ACSM's Guidelines for Exercise Testing and Prescription. USA*: Lippincott, Williams and Wilkins.

Brittenham, D & Brittenham, G (1997) *Stronger Abs and Backs.* USA: Human Kinetics.

Department of Health. (2004). *Choosing Health: Making healthier choices easier.* London: Department of Health)

Department of Health (2005). *Choosing Activity: A Physical Activity Action Plan.* London: Department of Health.

Department of Health (1996) *Strategy Statement on Physical Activity.* London: Department of Health

Difiore, Judy (2003) *The Complete Guide to Postnatal Fitness.* London: A & C Black

Lawrence, D & Barnett, L (2006) *GP Referral.* London: A & C Black.

Lawrence, D (2006) *The Complete Guide to Exercising Away Stress.* London: A & C Black.

Lawrence, D (2004) *The Complete Guide to Exercise to Music.* London: A & C Black.

Norris, C (2001) 2nd edition. *Abdominal training. Enhancing Core stability.* London. A & C Black

Norris C (1994) *Flexibility, Principles & Practice.* UK: A & C Black

INDEX

Page numbers with t show tables.